DEADLY DISEASES AND EPIDEMICS

YELLOW FEVER

DEADLY DISEASES AND EPIDEMICS

YELLOW FEVER

Brian R. Shmaefsky, Ph.D.

CONSULTING EDITOR
Hilary Babcock, M.D., M.P.H.,
Infectious Diseases Division,
Washington University School of Medicine,
Medical Director of Occupational Health (Infectious Diseases),
Barnes-Jewish Hospital and St. Louis Children's Hospital

FOREWORD BY
David L. Heymann
World Health Organization

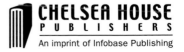
CHELSEA HOUSE
PUBLISHERS
An imprint of Infobase Publishing

Yellow Fever

Chelsea House
An imprint of Infobase Publishing
132 West 31st Street
New York NY 10001

Library of Congress Cataloging-in-Publication Data

Shmaefsky, Brian.
  Yellow fever / Brian R. Shmaefsky ; consulting editor, Hilary Babcock ; foreword by David L. Heymann.
     p. cm. — (Deadly diseases and epidemics)
  Includes bibliographical references and index.
  ISBN-13: 978-1-60413-231-1 (hardcover : alk. paper)
  ISBN-10: 1-60413-231-0 (hardcover : alk. paper) 1. Yellow fever—Juvenile literature. 2. Epidemics—Juvenile literature. I. Title.
  RA644.Y4S56 2010
  614.5'41—dc22
                    2009022328

Chelsea House books are available at special discounts when purchased in bulk quantities for businesses, associations, institutions, or sales promotions. Please call our Special Sales Department in New York at (212) 967-8800 or (800) 322-8755.

You can find Chelsea House on the World Wide Web at http://www.chelseahouse.com

Text design by Terry Mallon
Cover design by Takeshi Takahashi

Printed in the United States of America

Bang MSRF 10 9 8 7 6 5 4 3 2 1

This book is printed on acid-free paper.

All links and Web addresses were checked and verified to be correct at the time of publication. Because of the dynamic nature of the Web, some addresses and links may have changed since publication and may no longer be valid.

Table of Contents

Foreword

Communicable diseases kill and cause long-term disability. The microbial agents that cause them are dynamic, changeable, and resilient: They are responsible for more than 14 million deaths each year, mainly in developing countries.

Approximately 46 percent of all deaths in the developing world are due to communicable diseases, and almost 90 percent of these deaths are from AIDS, tuberculosis, malaria, and acute diarrheal and respiratory infections of children. In addition to causing great human suffering, these high-mortality communicable diseases have become major obstacles to economic development. They are a challenge to control either because of the lack of effective vaccines, or because the drugs that are used to treat them are becoming less effective because of antimicrobial drug resistance.

Millions of people, especially those who are poor and living in developing countries, are also at risk from disabling communicable diseases such as polio, leprosy, lymphatic filariasis, and onchocerciasis. In addition to human suffering and permanent disability, these communicable diseases create an economic burden—both on the workforce that handicapped persons are unable to join, and on their families and society, upon which they must often depend for economic support.

Finally, the entire world is at risk of the unexpected communicable diseases, those that are called emerging or reemerging infections. Infection is often unpredictable because risk factors for transmission are not understood, or because it often results from organisms that cross the species barrier from animals to humans. The cause is often viral, such as Ebola and Marburg hemorrhagic fevers and severe acute respiratory syndrome (SARS). In addition to causing human suffering and death, these infections place health workers at great risk and are costly to economies. Infections such as Bovine Spongiform Encephalopathy (BSE) and the associated new human variant of Creutzfeldt-Jakob Disease (vCJD) in Europe, and avian influenza A (H5N1) in Asia, are reminders of the seriousness of emerging and reemerging infections. In addition, many of these infections have the potential to cause pandemics, which are a constant threat to our economies and public health security.

Science has given us vaccines and anti-infective drugs that have helped keep infectious diseases under control. Nothing demonstrates the effectiveness of vaccines better than the successful eradication of smallpox, the decrease in polio as the eradication program continues, and the decrease in measles when routine immunization programs are supplemented by mass vaccination campaigns.

Likewise, the effectiveness of anti-infective drugs is clearly demonstrated through prolonged life or better health in those infected with viral diseases such as AIDS, parasitic infections such as malaria, and bacterial infections such as tuberculosis and pneumococcal pneumonia.

But current research and development is not filling the pipeline for new anti-infective drugs as rapidly as resistance is developing, nor is vaccine development providing vaccines for some of the most common and lethal communicable diseases. At the same time, providing people with access to existing anti-infective drugs, vaccines, and goods such as condoms or bed nets—necessary for the control of communicable diseases in many developing countries—remains a great challenge.

Education, experimentation, and the discoveries that grow from them are the tools needed to combat high mortality infectious diseases, diseases that cause disability, or emerging and reemerging infectious diseases. At the same time, partnerships between developing and industrialized countries can overcome many of the challenges of access to goods and technologies. This book may inspire its readers to set out on the path of drug and vaccine development, or on the path to discovering better public health technologies by applying our current understanding of the human genome and those of various infectious agents. Readers may likewise be inspired to help ensure wider access to those protective goods and technologies. Such inspiration, with pragmatic action, will keep us on the winning side of the struggle against communicable diseases.

David L. Heymann
Assistant Director General
Health Security and Environment
Representative of the Director General for Polio Eradication
World Health Organization
Geneva, Switzerland

1

The Yellow Fever Disease

The front-page headline was "The Fatal Yellow Plague." Underneath the headline was written, "Its ravages at New-Orleans. Ninety-five Deaths Reported Yesterday, the Fever Raging in an Infant Asylum. What The Young Men's Christian Association Is Doing." This story appeared in the New York Times *on September 8, 1878. Yellow fever was not supposed to be a fatal disease in the United States. It was a disease primarily of Central America, Cuba, and South America. On the day of the article, 232 were infected in New Orleans and 77 deaths were attributed to the yellow fever outbreak. Unfortunately, the disease was reported to have spread to 40 young children in Saint Vincent's Infant Asylum in New Orleans, which was run by a group called the Sisters of Charity.*

The news reported that the asylum was home to 200 babies of different nationalities. Concerns were raised in the news story that the cost of treating the outbreak was depleting the resources of the organization running the asylum. Organizations such as the Young Men's Christian Association were scrutinized by the news for their effectiveness at helping the children in the asylum. Aid was sought from the federal government including the U.S. War Office. A large effort involving many government agencies ensured that the children in the asylum received ample supplies of blankets, food, and medicine to deal with the rapidly spreading plague. The news story received day-by-day coverage in the New York Times *until the outbreak died down. It was stressed in news that yellow fever killed the young and the old, the rich and the poor, and did not discriminate by national origin, race, or religious affiliation.*[1]

A VIRAL DISEASE

Yellow fever is one of many human diseases caused by **microorganisms** called **viruses**. Viruses are generally defined as **infectious** particles that replicate only within the **cells** of other organisms. They typically are not classified with other organisms because viruses do not have a cell structure and do not possess most of the characteristics associated with being alive. A virus's structure is categorized as a **particle**, meaning that it is composed of simple chemical components. Viruses use the resources of their

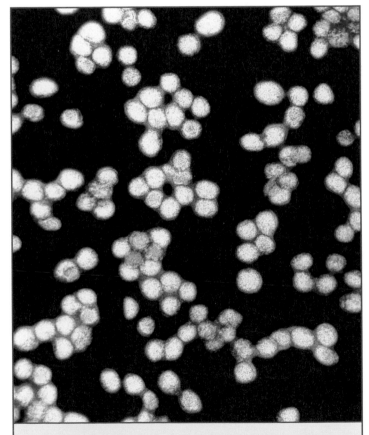

Figure 1.1 Yellow fever virus. (© Scientific/CDC/Visuals Unlimited, Inc.)

hosts to replicate, usually causing some type of harm as they carry out their **life cycle**. Because they cause harm, viruses are classified as **pathogens** or **parasites** by biologists.

Viruses have very simple lives that are carried out in a host's cells. Their life cycles involve going from one host to another, replicating in the host cells. The host can be an animal, a microorganism, or a plant. There is no typical way that viruses are transported from one host to another. Viruses can be directly or indirectly transmitted to a host. Direct transmission involves transfer of the virus by contact with body surfaces or body fluids. The **flu**, caused by the influenza virus, is spread through fluids sprayed out during coughing. In contrast, yellow fever is spread indirectly. It requires something called a **vector** to spread from one organism to another. Vectors are organisms or objects that pass a disease between organisms. The vector for yellow fever is a mosquito. Only certain types of mosquitoes can transmit the yellow fever virus. The virus must be able to survive long enough in the mosquito to be transmitted when the mosquito bites a human.

Most viruses live in a specific group of hosts called a *host range*. The yellow fever virus has a moderately narrow host range and is known to infect humans, monkeys, and other **primates**. In contrast, the **rabies** virus has a wide host range and can cause disease in bats, cats, coyotes, dogs, foxes, horses, humans, skunks, rabbits, raccoons, and rodents. Viruses also typically invade specific body cells in the host. For example, the highly specific **adenovirus**, one of the cold viruses, only attacks cells of the upper respiratory system. The yellow fever virus can attack almost any body cell in all of the body's **organ** systems. The ability of the virus to bind to certain types of **proteins** on the surface of cells results in the range of hosts and the specificity of body cells. Cells of different organisms have slightly dissimilar proteins. This is also true for proteins on the surfaces of different cells in the body. Apparently, the yellow fever virus can bind to a variety of protein types on the surfaces of body cells.

Viral diseases such as yellow fever are very difficult to control and eradicate. Attempts to exterminate the virus from the human population only lead to frustration. The virus is able to survive in wild animals, where it is picked up by mosquitoes and once again introduced to the human population. This was learned through the eradication of diseases such as **malaria** and **sleeping sickness.** Malaria and sleeping sickness are common diseases in tropical regions. Both of these diseases are spread by biting insects and are caused by microscopic organisms related to both animals and plants.

WHAT IS YELLOW FEVER?

Many types of disease organisms cause **fever** during an infection. Fever is an elevated body temperature response found in many types of infection or body damage. Yellow fever is one of a large assortment of viral fever diseases found in animals and humans. These diseases are mostly recognized by a prominent fever response of very high body temperatures ranging from 103 to 105°F (39.4 to 40.5°C). Normal body temperature averages 98.6°F (37°C). Yellow fever belongs to a category called vector-borne viral fevers because these illnesses are spread by agents that transfer the virus from one host to another.

Most medical professionals refer to yellow fever as **viral hemorrhagic fever,** or VHF. This places it in a category of related viral diseases noted for their ability to damage many body organs. All viral hemorrhagic fevers are **zoonotic** diseases, meaning that they can be spread from animals to humans. Examples of other viral hemorrhagic fevers are Ebola and Lassa, both discovered in Africa, and Marburg, named after the first identified outbreak in Germany.

Yellow fever gets its name from the fact that the disease typically causes the skin to yellow as well as producing a fever. Skin yellowing is due to a condition called **jaundice** that results from liver damage caused by the viral infection. If untreated, jaundice can lead to kidney failure and damage to the **central nervous system.** Many other viral diseases cause

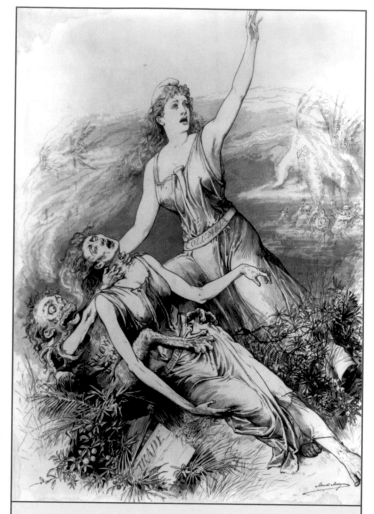

Figure 1.2 Editorial cartoon of "Yellow Jack," dragging Florida into the ground. (Library of Congress)

these conditions, making it difficult to identify yellow fever in patients.

Yellow fever is also known by other names. Throughout history yellow fever was called black vomit, vomito negro, sylvatic fever, and Yellow Jack. Black vomit, or vomito negro, refers to the very dark vomit that many infected people produce. Sylvatic fever gets is name from the observation that the disease is common in areas with many trees, such as a jungle. The name Yellow Jack was coined by the newspapers because yellow fever was perceived to be as destructive as any enemy troop. Cartoons depicted it as a skeleton wearing a yellow military jacket.

Yellow fever is generally classified into three major types, all having the same signs and symptoms: intermediate yellow fever, jungle yellow fever, and urban yellow fever. Intermediate yellow fever is found in humid grassland areas and is believed to be spread by mosquitoes that spread it from monkeys to humans. Jungle yellow fever occurs in rural areas where it is spread from human to human by mosquitoes found mostly in tropical jungles. Urban yellow fever is found in cities where it is transmitted from one human to another by mosquitoes living in small bodies of water around houses, other types of buildings, and fields. The diseases are indistinguishable and may overlap in areas where the different mosquitoes reside.

HISTORY OF YELLOW FEVER

Yellow fever is an ancient human disease that plagued societies before people fully understood the causes of infectious disease. Early civilizations did not know about **genetics, hygiene**, or microorganisms, so they were unaware of the major causes of disease. It is likely that they attributed disease to misfortune or some act of ill fate brought about by a deity. In early history, yellow fever was undoubtedly confused with other fever diseases. Any documentation of the disease before the 1700s was inaccurate for two reasons: confusion of the disease with other common ailments and a lack of knowledge of the disease by medical professionals. Early Egyptian medical documents show evidence of many diseases that fit the description of yellow fever.[2] These medical records gave accurate descriptions of the diseases. However, the descriptions overlapped with other diseases of the time, and they attributed disease to supernatural events.

The first accurate report of yellow fever was reported in the Yucatan, Mexico, in 1648, when many people came down with a condition that best matches yellow fever. It was believed that the disease made its way to Mexico from the Bahamas after people reported a similar disease that spread throughout the Caribbean islands. At first, the disease was most severe in the European settlers and was rare among the Africans brought to the Americas and Caribbean as slaves.

According to a description of the illness as seen among people involved in capturing and transporting African slaves during the American and European slave trade, "Not only would the patient's eyes turn watery and yellow, but the whole face would change, appearing 'unnatural,' denoting 'anxiety' and 'dejection of mind.'" Finally, it produced delirium and sometimes madness. During its progress, doctors noted changes "in the great mass of blood itself," which became putrefied and then oozed from the gums, nose, ears, and anus. The skin turned from flush to yellow or light brown. But it was in the final stages that patients underwent the worst of all symptoms: the black vomit, described variously by medical experts as resembling coffee grounds, black sand, kennel water, soot, or the meconium of newborn children.[3]

From the middle 1600s through the 1800s, yellow fever was identified in many coastal areas of Europe, South American, and North America. It started to evolve into a disease of all people. However, many physicians observed that it was less serious in people of African descent.

The spread of yellow fever was a mystery until the late 1880s. It was noted by medical professionals that yellow fever seemed to be prevalent in areas high in malaria. Malaria is one of the most common and deadly of the **protist** diseases. Yellow fever and malaria did not appear to be contagious through person-to-person contact, as with other infectious diseases. They were thought to spread by certain vapors given off by water or by contact with water. This was believed because these diseases were prevalent around bodies of water.

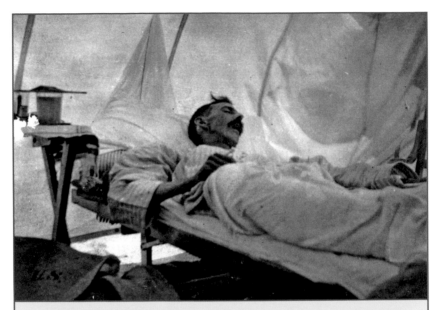

Figure 1.3 Patient suffering from yellow fever in Cuba, 1898, where during the Spanish-American War thousands died from the disease. (National Library of Medicine)

The first attempt to identify the spread of yellow fever was made in 1881, by Cuban scientist Carlos Finlay. This was in response to the large number of deaths from yellow fever that spread throughout the lower Mississippi valley in 1879. Finlay believed that a common mosquito of the tropical regions transmitted the disease through its bites. He concluded this because this type of mosquito was prevalent in areas with yellow fever, and because mosquitoes live in the same bodies of water where the disease is prevalent. Unfortunately, he could not perform any experiments to support his hypothesis. Any experimentation would have to involve infecting people with the potentially fatal disease.

Pressure to find the cause of yellow fever was fueled by the Spanish-American War, which took place in Cuba and Puerto Rico in 1898. More soldiers were dying from yellow fever than from war-related injuries. The Surgeon General of the United

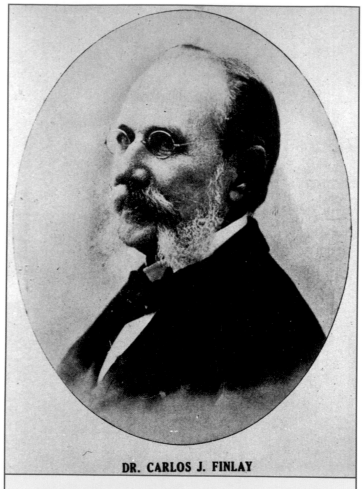

DR. CARLOS J. FINLAY

Figure 1.4 Cuban scientist Carlos Finlay, who in 1881 was the first to attempt to identify yellow fever, as many were dying from the disease. He was the first to hypothesize that mosquitoes spread the disease. (National Library of Medicine)

States assembled a group of medical researchers to find the cause of yellow fever. This effort was led by army surgeon Walter Reed. He was assisted by surgeons Aristides Agramonte, James Carroll, and Jesse Lazear. They evaluated many ideas about disease spread, including the hypothesis by Carlos Finlay.

Reed's team conducted an experiment using military volunteers. They first tested whether the disease was spread through direct contact by having volunteers sleep on bedding and clothing from yellow fever patients. The volunteers were kept in a room in which no possible vectors can enter. This experiment showed that yellow fever was not transmitted that way when none of the volunteers developed the disease. In another experiment, Reed's team isolated a group of volunteers and exposed them to mosquitoes that were fed on people infected with yellow

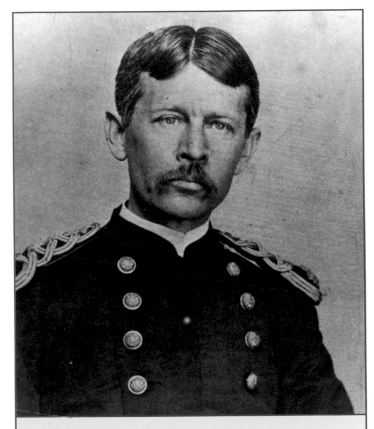

Figure 1.5 U.S. Army surgeon Walter Reed and his research team in 1901 confirmed the hypothesis that the Aedes aegypti mosquito spread the yellow fever virus. (National Library of Medicine)

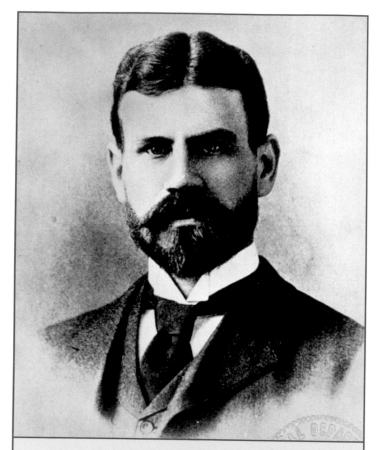

Figure 1.6 American physician Jesse William Lazear, one of Reed's team of researchers, died at 34 years of age from yellow fever, and was later believed to have experimented on himself. (National Library of Medicine)

fever. The volunteers contracted the yellow fever, supporting the idea that it was spread by mosquito bites.

Reed's human experiments gained criticism from the scientific community because it intentionally exposed healthy subjects to a deadly disease. Reed believed that Jesse Lazear subsequently experimented on himself, leading to his death from yellow fever in 1900. Lazear's laboratory notebooks hinted at self-experimentation. Just before his death, Lazear wrote in letter to his wife, "I rather think I am on the track of the real germ." This was the last letter written by Lazear, who died 17 days later. It was speculated that other people working in Reed's laboratory also died from intentional exposure. In spite of the controversy, Major William Gorgas performed a mosquito eradication program in Cuba that significantly reduced the spread of yellow fever in Cuba by the early 1900s.

Public health officials in the early 1900s hypothesized that yellow fever originated in Africa and was imported into other areas with the slave trade. An article written by Rubert Boyce in the 1910 *British Medical Journal* led him to believe that yellow fever was native to West Africa.[4] He based his findings on studies showing that native people of West Africa developed a less severe form of the disease. It was hypothesized that they adapted to the disease over time and that their bodies were able to fight off the viral infection. Later studies on the **immune system** confirmed his findings.

The research on yellow fever helped with the discovery of the spread of malaria in 1897. British medical officer Ronald Ross showed that the protist causing malaria was likely transmitted to people by mosquitoes. He used a disease called bird malaria as a model for studying human transmission. Ross's work was confirmed by Italian scientist Giovanni Batista Grassi in 1899. It was also concluded that mosquito control would stop the spread of malaria as it did for yellow fever.

Today, it is not unusual to use mosquito control as the primary strategy for reducing the spread of diseases carried by mosquitoes. Many countries have comprehensive mosquito control measures using guidelines established by the **Centers for Disease Control and Prevention** in the United States and by the **World Health Organization** of the **United Nations. Vaccination** programs are globally encouraged to prevent the occurrence of yellow fever in areas where mosquito control is not fully effective. Yellow fever is now considered a rare disease, whereas, in the 1900s, it was on the verge of becoming a major plague of warm regions across the globe.

2

Viral Diseases

To many tourists, Brazil is an exotic travel location known for delicious churrasco (barbeque), pristine beaches, tropical rain forests, and vibrant entertainment. However, few travelers who vacation in Brazil are familiar with the many infectious viral diseases that plague the country. Yellow fever is one of the viral diseases found throughout Brazil. On January 8, 2008, the Brazilian Ministry of Health confirmed 45 cases of yellow fever between December 2007 and the date of their report. Physicians reported 25 deaths among these cases. Usually, no more than 35 cases of yellow fever a year occur in Brazil. Panic spread through the major cities of Brazil as people began seeking medical advice. Physicians' offices and hospitals were crowded with people requesting yellow fever vaccination.

Much of the panic occurred in urban areas of Brazil. Yet, most of the cases were found in rural regions around the Amazon River in the northern part of the country (Figure 2.1). This region has many bodies of water where the mosquitoes that carry yellow fever thrive. Public health officials had to quell the panic by educating people about the unlikely spread of the mosquitoes to the urban regions hundred of miles away from the outbreak.

Brazil accounts for roughly 25 percent of the yellow fever cases in South America. Neighboring countries such as Argentina and Venezuela had heightened yellow fever alerts as a result of the outbreak in Brazil. Each country sent out public statements encouraging people to reduce exposure to mosquitoes and to remove items outdoors that could collect water and harbor mosquitoes. Vaccinations were recommended in urban areas close to the outbreak.[1]

VIRAL STRUCTURE AND CLASSIFICATION

Ancient people suffered from a variety of viral diseases long before viruses were discovered as disease agents. Egyptian hieroglyphs from approximately

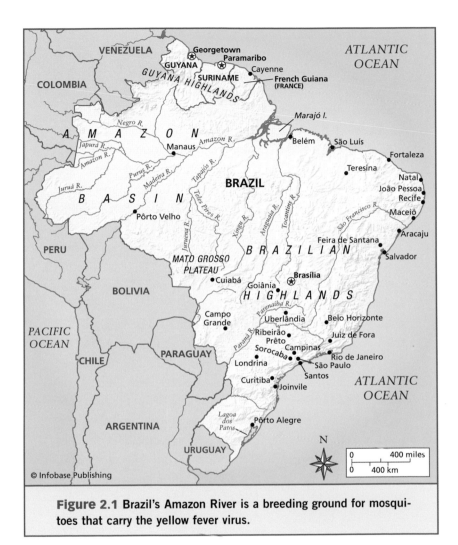

Figure 2.1 Brazil's Amazon River is a breeding ground for mosquitoes that carry the yellow fever virus.

3700 B.C. recorded evidence of the viral disease **poliomyelitis** or polio, which was discovered by Dr. Karl Landsteiner in 1909. Medical researchers studying the mummy of Pharaoh Ramses V, who died in 1196 B.C., discovered scarring on the dried skin of his face and body that was consistent with the viral disease **smallpox**.

The discovery of viruses as a unique life form came about in 1892. Dmitri Iwanowski, a Russian botanist, accidentally revealed that viruses were responsible for a common tobacco disease. He determined this by **filtering** the diseased **tissues** in an attempt to collect the organism causing the tobacco disease. Iwanowski was amazed when he discovered that the disease organism was smaller than any known cell. Other scientists carried out similar studies on other diseases and called the disease organisms "unfilterable infectious **agents.**" This filtration method distinguished viruses from bacterial, fungal, and protistan diseases, which did not pass through filters. These unfilterable agents were renamed in 1915. Scientists generally used the term *Twort particles* for viruses causing agricultural animal disease, named after English biologist Frederick William Twort, who isolated viruses from cattle.

It is not known when the term *virus* replaced *Twort particles.* At the time viruses were named Twort particles, the term *virus* was used to describe any infectious agent, as had been established by the medical community since 1729. The original meaning of *virus,* "venomous substances," originated in 1392. In 1729, the term *virus* was restricted to living venoms. The adjective form "viral" was used in the scientific literature in 1948. Physicians and scientists use a similar term, **virulent,** when describing aggressive diseases caused by any microorganism. Virulent means extremely infectious or poisonous. It dates back to the Latin word *virulentus,* which means poisonous.

Viruses belong to a simple group of microscopic living entities called *particles.* Their structure and function is too simple to classify with other living organisms because they lack most of the living properties of other creatures. In addition, they are so small that they must be viewed with powerful **electron microscopes** that magnify the virus to one million times. Scientists generally categorize particles into **prions, viroids,** viruses, and **virusoids.**

Prions are the simplest of the infectious particles. They are composed only of protein and somehow induce the host cell to convert its proteins into the prion protein. Prions are responsible for **mad cow disease** and **Creutzfeldt-Jakob Disease (CJD)**. Viroids are composed of a single strand of **nucleic acid** called **ribonucleic acid (RNA)**. They use the host cell's chemistry to manufacture copies of the viroid RNA. They most commonly cause diseases in plants. Viruses are typically made up of a piece of genetic material surrounded by a protein capsule. Their replication induces the cell to assemble the virus particle using the cell's chemistry. Virusoids are similar to viroids except they require the presence of a virus in order to replicate in a cell. This virus is called a helper virus because it assists with the replication of the virusoid. They cause disease in a variety of organisms.

Little was known about the structure of viruses until a technique called **crystallography** was used to determine the chemical composition of viruses. Crystallography was developed in 1912 by German physicist Max von Laue. The technique uses X-rays to determine the shapes of large **molecules**. Crystallography studies determined that viruses were a combination of nucleic acids and proteins. Another technique called transmission electron microscopy was used to determine the structure of a virus by German physician Helmuth Ruska in 1940. He confirmed that a virus has no cell structure and resembles a simple assemblage of molecules. It was later proposed that viruses were made of a core of nucleic acids encased in a shell made of proteins.

Only a few common plant viruses were available for study in the early years of **virology**. Scientists generalized the information on these viruses to come up with a model of a representative virus. However, scientists have since discovered that there is no typical virus. Scientists have shown through years of experimentation that viruses are typically composed of nucleic acid genetic material enclosed in a protein casing (Figure 2.2) called a **capsid**. It is now known that viruses vary greatly in their chemical composition and the organization of their **genome,** or genetic material. In addition, there is great variability in the structure of the capsid.

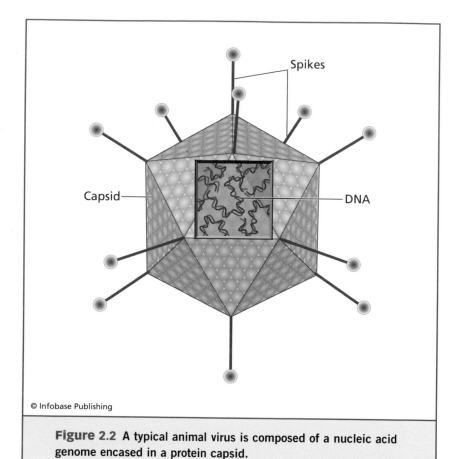

Figure 2.2 A typical animal virus is composed of a nucleic acid genome encased in a protein capsid.

A virus's genome can be composed of **deoxyribonucleic acid (DNA)** or RNA. All other known organisms contain DNA as their genetic material. RNA is usually used to assist with the function of DNA. The capsid is typically composed of protein units programmed in the virus's genome. Capsids come in a variety of shapes and sizes. The main function of the capsid is to protect the viral genome from environmental damage.

Various environmental conditions can damage the viral genome, including corrosive chemicals, **enzymes**, and ultra-violet light. Corrosive chemicals break apart or wear away materials gradually by chemical action. Many types of acids and bases can destroy the genome. Oxygen is also destructive to the genome because it changes the information contained in the DNA. Enzymes produced by **bacteria** and other organisms can break down unprotected viral genomes. Ultraviolet light is a high-energy light that can damage many types of molecules, including DNA and RNA. The viral capsid is capable of blocking corrosive chemicals and enzymes. Certain proteins in the capsid likely absorb the damaging effects of ultraviolet light.

The viral genome is composed of either DNA or RNA. The nucleic acid composition of the viral genome is a major factor in classifying viruses. **DNA viruses** possess DNA that is either double stranded or single stranded. **Double-stranded** DNA, made up of two chains of nucleic acids attached side by side, forms a typical double helix pattern (Figure 2.3). **Single-stranded** DNA is made up of only one chain of nucleic acids that is twisted upon itself to form a double helix. The strands of DNA viruses can be linear—in a straight line—or circular. Double-stranded circular DNA is the most stable form of DNA and is difficult to break down.

RNA viruses can also be double-stranded or single-stranded. Single-stranded RNA viruses can be classified as **positive-sense RNA** or **negative sense RNA**. The replication of negative-sense RNA viruses is very complex compared to DNA viruses and positive-sense RNA viruses. Double-stranded RNA viruses typically have the strands arranged into a double helix similar to the pattern found in DNA viruses. Single-stranded RNA viruses are usually looped into patterns in which segments of the nucleic acid chain overlap and combine. The helix formation and looping pattern protects the RNA from chemicals that degrade the single-strand structure.

A typical viral capsid is made up of similar protein units that lock together to form the casing. These units of proteins are generally called **capsomeres**. The suffix "mere" in capsomere means "a piece of" and refers to the units of protein. Some scientists spell capsomere as "capsomer." Capsomeres have two

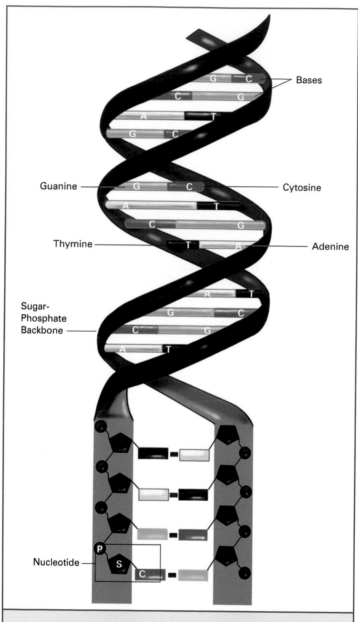

Figure 2.3 DNA viruses contain either one or two strands of DNA twisted into a helix. (National Institute of General Medical Sciences)

unique features that assist viral replication. One feature is that the capsomeres lock together to form structures in a manner similar to LEGO bricks. The shape and arrangement of capsomeres can produce a specific form of capsid. Most viruses are composed of identical capsomeres that form the final capsid shape. A second feature is that capsomeres are self assembling, which means that they can form complex structures on their own by attaching to each other or to other chemicals. This means that the host cell does not need to build the capsomeres into the capsid.

Aside from the capsomeres, capsids contain other types of proteins. Many of these proteins are needed to help the virus complete its life cycle. One group of proteins is commonly called virus **attachment proteins.** At first scientists called these proteins **antigens.** An antigen is any substance that can produce an **immune response**—a set of reactions the body uses to attack and remove foreign substances that enter the body. Antigens were discovered by American biologist George Hirst in 1941. Hirst detected viral antigens when he noticed blood attacking the viral antigen as part of an immune response. Attachment proteins help viruses locate and attach themselves to specific types of cells. They also assist with the virus's ability to enter a host cell. The uniqueness of attachment proteins determines the types of organisms and cells a virus can invade.

Capsids for most viruses are shaped like boxes and spirals. Certain types of viruses have complex forms that take on strikingly unique shapes. For example, viruses called **bacteriophages** resemble small machines with legs designed to land on a cell and a needle intended to inject the viral genome into the cell. Some viruses have an inner capsid attached to the genome. This structure is called a **nucleocapsid.** Nucleocapsid proteins are different from the capsid proteins and self-assemble around the viral genome, forming an inner casing over the genetic material. Research studies show that the nucleocapsid stabilizes the genome of viruses with a fragile form of genetic material.

Nucleocapsids are typically found in viruses with certain forms of DNA and RNA that are unstable and readily decay.

Certain viruses have a capsid surrounded by an **envelope**. An envelope is a structure resembling a **cell membrane**. The cell membrane is a layer of fat and protein that encompasses a cell and holds in the cell contents. Viruses that possess this covering are called **enveloped viruses**. Scientists use the term *naked virus* to explain viruses lacking an envelope. The envelope is made of components from the infected cell and virus capsid. Enveloped viruses acquire part of the cell membrane when they exit the infected cell after replicating. The virus then places the attachment proteins and other types of protein into the envelope. Research studies show the envelope has two major functions: It protects the virus from drying and is a barrier against enzymes capable of breaking down proteins and nucleic acids. The envelope also assists the virus in entering host cells. Certain enveloped viruses contain enzymes that help the virus quickly take over the cells that they invade.

VIRAL LIFE CYCLES

A classic study from 1952, called the Hershey-Chase blender experiment, used a viral life cycle to confirm that nucleic acids were the genetic material of organisms. They used radioactive labels to trace the movement of the DNA and capsid after the viruses were introduced to bacterial cultures. At the time of the experiment, scientists believed that DNA was the only type of nucleic acid that carried the genetic information. From this experiment they learned that DNA is the component of the virus that causes disease in the cells and is involved in viral replication. Now it is known that RNA and even proteins can convey inheritable information.

The life of a virus requires the resources of a host cell. A host provides all the cell components needed for the virus to make copies of itself. The virus's simple structure does not contain the components needed for self-replication. Scientists use this type of relationship in defining viruses as **intracellular** parasites. Intracellular means something that takes place within the cell. Viruses use the **metabolism** of a host to build new viruses. The virus merely provides the blueprint for constructing the virus. Unfortunately for the host cell, it expends much of the energy it needs to stay alive constructing multiple copies of the virus. In most cases, the host cell dies as of a result of the viral replication. Death can be due either to disruption of the cell's metabolism or to destruction of the cell by the body's immune system. The body tries to reduce replication of the virus by killing infected cells.

Viruses generally bring about disease because they must infect cells of other organisms in order to replicate. A virus does not reproduce like other organisms. Most other organisms carry out cell division to replicate cells or make **gametes** for sexual reproduction. The virus reproduces by providing the host cells with a blueprint for building multiple copies of the virus. This blueprint is written into the viral DNA, which contains the genetic information to make copies of the capsomeres, genome, and other capsid proteins. The virus uses the host cell's metabolism to manufacture viral components. The virus's genome carries just enough information to take control of the host cell and direct the cell to replicate the virus.

Viruses have no ability to maintain their structure and replicate when outside of a host cell. Almost all viruses must be able to find a host cell before the capsid breaks down and the genome decays. Dehydration, enzymes, sunlight, and corrosive chemicals in the environment can damage the capsid, which protects the genome from being degraded. The time a virus can sit intact in the environment varies greatly by type of virus and environmental conditions. Double-stranded genomes are very stable and persist when viruses are not in a host. However, they are usually degraded by long exposure to corrosive chemicals, enzymes from body fluids and microorganisms, and sunlight. Single-stranded genomes are unstable and decay naturally over time. Under favorable environmental conditions some viruses are inactivated after several hours while others may remain intact for days. Viruses can remain undamaged for decades in continuously frozen environments sheltered from the sun.

Most viruses require seven events for replication in a host cell. These events result in the production of hundreds to thousands of replicated viruses. The stages vary in complexity based on the structure of the capsid and the composition of a virus's genome. The first stage of the viral life cycle is **transmission** to a host cell. Transmission is defined as the passing of a disease organism from an infected organism to one that is not infected with the disease. The transmission stage is critical because the virus must make it to a new host organism before the virus is damaged to the point that it cannot replicate.

Viruses completely rely on the environment or the host organism to carry out the means of transmission. For many viruses, some activity of the host organism directly transfers the virus to another organism. The activity encourages the virus to leave the body where it can then make contact with another host. Certain viruses are transmitted to a new host by a vector. In complex animals and plants, viruses must be transmitted from cell to cell within the body as well as being transferred to a new host. Successful transmission means that the virus must make contact with uninfected host cell. For most viruses this means that the virus must enter the body and be transferred somehow to the particular cells that they infect. For example, the meningitis virus must be able to reach the nervous system in order to replicate.

Successful transmission of the virus leads to the second stage: **adsorption**. Adsorption means to stick onto something. The adsorption stage of viral infection involves attachment to the host cell surface. Adsorption typically occurs on particular cells of the host. Attachment takes place when viruses come across a cell that has cell membrane **receptors** that selectively bind to the viral attachment proteins. A receptor is a protein that binds to a specific chemical. There are many types of receptors found on the outer surface of the cell membrane. Receptors carry out a diversity of functions for the cell including the detection of certain chemicals such as hormones. Viruses must attach to a specific receptor, yet they cannot seek it out. They are transmitted randomly to host cells and by chance may reach a cell that matches their attachment proteins.

After adsorption the viral infection progresses to the third stage, which is called **penetration**. Penetration is the process of entering into or through something. Naked viruses stimulate the cell to engulf or swallow the virus upon attachment to the correct receptor. Cells engulf viruses by covering the virus with a bubble of cell membrane. The cell then moves the bubble into the cell, swallowing up the virus. Enveloped viruses enter a cell by fusing with the cell membrane. Upon fusion, the virus either blends with the cell or is engulfed in a bubble of cell membrane. The virus is not yet active at this point of infection.

The fourth stage, **uncoating,** takes place after the host cell engulfs the virus. At this point, the virus becomes active. During the uncoating stage the virus envelope and capsid break apart, releasing the viral genome into the fluids within the cell. Viral replication cannot take place without exposure of the genome. The genome makes contact with the cell's metabolic enzymes in the **cytoplasm** at this stage. Researchers have discovered that once the virus it uncoated it is very difficult to find the viral genome in the host cell. Scientists call this the eclipse phase because it seems that the virus is hiding in the cell. At the uncoating stage it is possible for the host cell to destroy the virus by using enzymes and other molecules designed to ward off viral attack.

Following the uncoating stage is the fifth stage: synthesis. At this stage the host cell is directed by the virus to replicate the viral genome and capsomeres. The synthesis stage varies greatly, as each virus has a specific synthesis stage based on its genome composition and type of capsid. The viral genome serves as the blueprint for building the viral components. Many viruses start the synthesis stage by first producing **repressor proteins** that control certain host cell functions. The virus overrides many of the cell activities when building new viruses. At this point, the cell is not functioning normally and does not carry out many vital functions. Some cells die prematurely at this stage and in turn stop viral replication. In humans, infected cells usually release chemicals that initiate an immune response targeted at controlling viral replication. This also leads to death of the infected cell.

The sixth stage of viral infection is called the assembly stage. It is sometimes called the **maturation phase** because the viral components are maturing into a complete virus. During assembly the viral parts come together to form new viruses. Multiple copies of new genomes are made using the cell's chemistry for making replica viral DNA and RNA from nucleic acid or **nucleotide** building blocks in the cell. The copies of the genome then bind to viral proteins, combining the genome copies with many capsomeres. The replicated capsomere proteins self-assemble around the genome or the nucleocapsid. Other proteins are also made by the host cell and self-assemble into the capsid structure. Many of the mature viruses contain defects, including incomplete genomes and abnormal capsids. The number of defective viruses is insignificant compared to the number of normal viruses that will move along successfully to the last stage of viral infection.

The final event of the viral life cycle is the release stage. Like the synthesis stage, this stage varies greatly between different types of viruses. Certain viruses are released from the cell by programming it to undergo **lysis**—breakdown and subsequent death of a cell. The systematic programmed death of a cell is called **apoptosis**. A cell can be stimulated to lyse by specific viral proteins. In many cases a cell will gradually undergo lysis as it slowly dies during the viral infection. Certain viruses will remain in the cell for long periods of time without going through a release phase. They may release later depending on various conditions of the host body or the environment. In certain cases these delayed viruses can cause a cell to replicate rapidly and produce a tumor. It is possible for some tumors to develop into cancer, as in **cervical cancer**.

Enveloped viruses usually bud from the cell during the release stage. A bud is a small protrusion of the cell membrane. The virus forms a bud by being pushed against the inner surface of the cell until it becomes enveloped in an outward bubble of cell membrane. The bud is then released, and this produces a viral capsid surrounded by the envelope. Viral proteins are sometimes inserted into the envelope before the virus buds from the cell. These enzymes assist with the virus's assembly stage. Enveloped viruses do not necessarily induce apoptosis. Many of them bud slowly keeping the cell alive for the natural lifetime of the cell. This situation produces a persistent infection that results in a long illness.

The sickness and body damage associated with a viral infection is usually due to a loss of cell function. Other problems are likely due to side effects of the immune response to the virus. Viral replication prevents cells from carrying out critical tasks needed by a particular part of the body. Some of these cell functions may affect how the whole body functions. The time it takes to feel ill depends on the speed of viral replication. A certain number of cells must be infected before the body is affected by nonfunctioning cells. In addition, the intensity of the immune response increases as more viruses populate the body. Viruses that infect cells of critical body organs can produce severe effects on the body and can lead to death. Other problems created by viral infections are caused by the immune system. Many viruses cause the immune system to release chemicals that produce fever, a runny nose, rashes, tiredness, and watery eyes. Various other chemicals can accidentally kill healthy cells.

THE YELLOW FEVER VIRUS

The yellow fever virus belongs to a family of viruses called *Flaviviridae*, which belongs to a large grouping of viruses called the togaviruses. This family of viruses gets it name from the Latin term *flavus*, which means "yellow." Flaviviruses primarily cause disease in humans and cattle. However, these viruses can live in a variety of insects and **mammals**. There are three major categories of flaviviruses: Flavivirus, Pestivirus, and Hepacivirus. Flavivirus causes yellow fever, Pestivirus produces diarrhea in cattle, and Hepacivirus attacks the liver of humans. The yellow fever virus is related to various modern plague viruses such as **dengue fever, hepatitis G, St. Louis encephalitis,** and **West Nile disease**. Like yellow fever, they are spread by mosquitoes and biting flies.

All viruses are given a number by the **International Committee on Taxonomy of Viruses** (ICTV), which further classifies viruses into an individual type.[2] This classification system is called the ICTVdB Virus Code. The virus code for the yellow fever virus is Virus Code: 00.026.0.01.001. The **National Institutes of Health** places the yellow fever virus into a grouping called the NCBI Taxon Identifier Taxonomy ID: 11089. ID 11089 refers to a group of 10 genetically different flaviviruses that cause different types of yellow fever in humans. The types of yellow fever virus are called: YFV 17D, YFV 1899/81; YFV isolate Angola/14FA/1971; YFV isolate Ethiopia/Couma/1961; YFV isolate Ivory Coast/1999; YFV isolate Ivory Coast/85-82H/1982; YFV isolate Uganda/A7094A4/1948; YFV strain French neurotropic vaccine; YFV strain Ghana/Asibi/1927; and YFV Trinidad/79A/1979.

The yellow fever virus genome is composed of a linear positive-sense, single-stranded RNA. Its RNA is made up of 11,000 nucleotides, which is much simpler than the human genome composed of 3 billion nucleotides. The yellow fever virus genome primarily programs for capsomere and attachment proteins. Because it is an RNA virus, a replication protein is also part of the genome to help the virus replicate.

Yellow fever is an enveloped virus with a spherical capsid (Figure 2.4). Attached to the genome is a nucleocapsid. The virus is 40 to 50 nanometers in diameter, meaning it takes 5 million viruses placed side by side to equal one inch. Its nucleocapsid is shaped like a box and is 25 to 30 nanometers

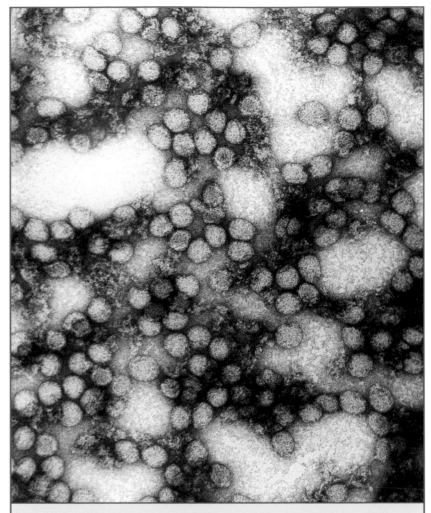

Figure 2.4 Yellow fever is an enveloped virus with a spherical capsid. (Centers for Disease Control and Prevention)

in diameter. The capsomere proteins are uniform and interlock to form the capsid. Nucleocapsid proteins intertwine with the RNA genome, forming a geometric pattern that fits snuggly into the capsid. Protein spikes that serve as attachment proteins are inserted onto the outer surface of envelope.

3

Disease Course and Epidemiology

Global climate change is of international concern, causing many countries to review energy use policies in an attempt to reduce carbon dioxide pollution. There are many ways global climate change may impact society if it is allowed to occur without constraint. Many scientists hypothesize that changes in weather from global climate change can affect agriculture in ways that could cause economic turmoil and famine. Scientists who study public health are concerned about the impact of changing temperatures on populations of insects that spread infectious disease such as yellow fever.

Ample research shows that warmer temperatures and increased rainfall can encourage the spread of mosquitoes into regions where they normally cannot thrive. Some areas of the United States, such as Houston, Texas, have seen tropical diseases appear with regularity. This is associated with the arrival and settlement of tropical insects that spread these diseases. Dengue fever, which is transmitted like yellow fever, is on the rise in Houston and other American cities bordering Mexico.[1]

Climate and its possible impact on public health is not a new issue. It has been recognized as a potential problem in the United States since 1840, when German pathologist Jacob Henle wrote in his 1840 treatise called *On Miasmata and Contagia,* "Heat and moisture favor the production and propagation of the infusoria and the molds, as well as the miasmata and contagia, therefore miasmatic-contagious diseases are most often endemic in warm moist regions and epidemic in the wet summer months." Changes in the distribution of yellow fever were one of the major concerns he mentioned with regard to climate.[2]

THE YELLOW FEVER VIRUS LIFE CYCLE

Unlike many viruses, the yellow fever virus is highly competent at invading multiple hosts and infecting a variety of cells within the host body. Scientists believe that yellow fever was naturally found in African monkeys long before it became a human disease. This is also the case for other human viral diseases such as AIDS and Ebola. Researchers noted that the accidental introduction of yellow fever into South America immediately caused illness in the local monkey populations. Ultimately, the disease took residence in monkeys throughout the tropical Latin American countries. Little is known about how monkeys initially contracted the virus, but it is known that related viruses are common in rats. Monkeys may have acquired the disease from rats tens of thousands of years ago.

Yellow fever spreads within the monkey population through the bites of bloodsucking insects. The same is true for how it is transmitted through the human population. Many viruses are transmitted by only one or a few types of biting insect vectors. Yellow fever has a broad range of vectors. The disease is commonly spread between humans by a **genus** of mosquitoes called *Aedes*. This genus of mosquitoes transmitted other types of diseases such as malaria. *Aedes aegypti, A. africanus, A. simpsoni, A. furcifer,* and *A. luteocephalus* transmit yellow fever throughout Africa. Most of these mosquitoes are found coast to coast in the central regions of northern Africa. *Aedes albopictus,* the Asian tiger mosquito, spreads yellow fever throughout Asia. Unintentional infection with yellow fever has occurred in laboratories and hospitals. This occurs through contact with blood and tissues from infected patients.

Currently, the spread of yellow fever in the Americas is carried out primarily by local mosquitoes. *Aedes* mosquitoes accidentally introduced from Africa and Asia also spread yellow fever in Central and South America. They were inadvertently transported by ship with the early slave trade and currently enter the Americas with cargo shipments on airplanes and ships. Urban yellow fever is spread by *A. aegypti,* which breeds in cities. Sylvatic yellow fever is transmitted by *Haemagogus* and *Mansoni* mosquitoes that live in the tops of the forests and jungles. Other insects such as biting flies (phlebotomine flies) spread yellow fever in South America. In addition, other **arthropods,** such as the tick, *Amblyomma variegatum,* transmit yellow fever in West Africa.

Arthropods contract the yellow fever virus when they suck the blood of an infected monkey or human. Most urban yellow fever is contracted from humans. Monkeys are a major source of yellow fever in forest and jungle regions. This is called the oral infectivity stage of the viral life cycle. The virus can only live in **competent** arthropods. Competency is the ability of a vector to harbor and spread a disease organism. It is known that the virus resides in the mosquito's body for two weeks before becoming

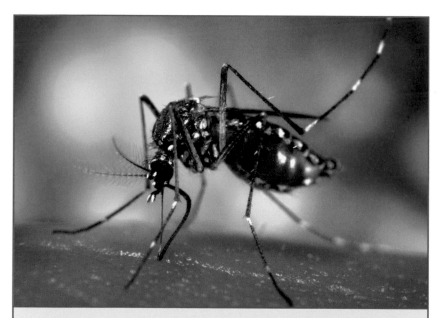

Figure 3.1 *Aedes egypti* is one of the major yellow fever vectors. The mosquito is native to Africa but has been unintentionally transported to many warmer regions in the world. (Centers for Disease Control and Prevention)

infectious. However, the virus begins replicating in the mosquito's body after three days. The virus first reproduces in cells in the mosquito's digestive system and fat cells. It then travels to the nervous system, **salivary glands**, and reproductive system. *Aedes* mosquitoes have a rapid life cycle. They can develop into young adult mosquitoes two weeks after the eggs are laid in water.

The virus is spread to a human or monkey when the virus escapes into the **saliva** that enters the host's body during the mosquito bite to initiate the virus's transition stage. Yellow fever viruses are also passed from a mosquito to its offspring through the mosquito eggs, giving rise to mosquitoes containing the virus at birth. This occurs because viruses in infected female mosquitoes travel from the reproductive system into the egg. The virus then enters the host replication stage of its life. Yellow fever viruses have two complete life cycles. One is carried out in the mosquito and the other in the monkey or human host.

A bite from an infected mosquito deposits viruses into the host's bloodstream. Once in the bloodstream, the virus must travel to host cells to replicate. This task is facilitated as the heart pumps the infected blood to every body organ. However, the virus is subject to attack by the immune system as it travels to its destination. The viruses cannot reproduce in the blood liquids. They must enter the cytoplasm of specific body cells. Viruses must first find and attach to certain host cell receptors to start the adsorption stage. The yellow fever virus normally binds to the nervous system cells of monkeys. In humans, the virus attacks **epithelial** cells. Epithelial cells are found in almost all major body organs and are found lining body cavities. The virus also attaches to receptors on heart cells. Certain types of yellow fever viruses, called **neurotropic** strains, can attack the human brain.

After attaching to the host cell, the viruses are taken into the cell and then uncoat, releasing their RNA genome from the capsid and nucleocapsid. The envelope is lost as the viruses enter the cell. It is most common for the virus to begin replicating in cells of the digestive and respiratory systems early in

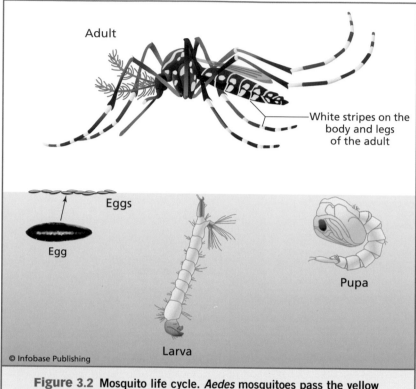

Adult

White stripes on the body and legs of the adult

Eggs

Egg

Pupa

Larva

© Infobase Publishing

Figure 3.2 Mosquito life cycle. *Aedes* mosquitoes pass the yellow fever virus to offspring through the mosquito eggs.

the infection. They have a high affinity for the epithelial cells of these organ systems. After uncoating, the yellow fever virus enters a combined replication and assembly stage.

The replication part of this stage of the yellow fever virus first involves an RNA synthesis phase. Viral RNA has two purposes in the host cell. The cell uses enzymes to construct a minus-strand RNA molecule, using the original viral RNA as a template to guide the synthesis of the virus's nucleic acid sequence. This minus-strand RNA molecule is then used by the cell to replicate copies of the virus's RNA genome. Scientists are still working out the mechanism of RNA replication of the yellow fever virus and other positive-strand RNA viruses. It is known that a section of the viral genome called a **promoter** initiates replication of the viral RNA. Recent research studies show that a promoter called the flavivirus RdRp promoter helps the virus make a minus-strand RNA.

The original positive-strand RNA is also used as a set of instructions for producing viral proteins such as the capsomeres and the attachment proteins. This overlaps with the final assembly part of the combined stage. New viruses are formed as the nucleocapsid starts to collect and envelop the viral RNA. The capsomere proteins then spontaneously build capsids around the newly formed nucleocapsids. Copies of the virus are continually made as new copies of the viral RNA are synthesized by the minus-strand RNA templates. The assembled viruses enter a cell structure called the **endoplasmic reticulum**. In the endoplasmic reticulum, the viruses are placed in small sacks that move the virus to the outer membrane of the cell. The viruses then bud out of the cell, poking an opening in the cell's outer membrane. Small pieces of this membrane and the transport sack then become the virus's envelope. This process of leaving the cell is called budding.

Newly created viruses can then travel through the blood or can attach to nearby uninfected cells. In many cases, the viruses start invading cells of the heart, kidneys, liver, and nervous system. The virus can only exit the body when the person is bitten by a bloodsucking insect. A certain amount of viruses must be in the blood for the insect to become contaminated with the virus. The disease is more likely to be spread to mosquitoes in a person who has an advanced case of yellow fever because the virus population is very high in their blood. The amount of virus is measured in a unit called the viral **titer**.

THE SCIENCE OF STUDYING DISEASES

Epidemiology is the study of the occurrence and frequency of a disease in a population of organisms. To effectively investigate a disease, **epidemiologists** need a thorough understanding of the causes, predisposing factors, and transmission of a particular disease. Epidemiology uses a variety of strategies that provide information into the spread and distribution of infectious diseases such as yellow fever. It may take many years to fully understand enough about an infectious disease to predict when and where it will strike in a population. The study of yellow fever involves epidemiological investigations typical to the study of infectious disease. Other fields of epidemiology investigate diseases due to genetic and environmental factors. Infectious diseases such as yellow fever have genetic and environmental factors that predispose a person to the disease.

Epidemiologists and physicians in the early days of epidemiology focused on the control of infectious deadly diseases that plagued their countries at the time. They developed ways to track the spread of organisms that caused infectious diseases in humans and agricultural animals. They also relied on the research of Robert Koch, who, in the late 1800s, developed strategies for identifying the causative agents of infectious diseases. He proposed four decisive factors for confirming whether a particular organism was the cause of a specific infectious disease. Koch's factors were: 1) the organism must be associated in every instance of the disease; 2) the organism must be extracted from the body and grown in a culture for several generations; 3) the disease could be reproduced in experimental animals through a pure culture; and 4) the organism could be retrieved from the inoculated animal and cultured again. Unfortunately, criteria 3 and 4 are not always easy to achieve. Some organisms, such as the yellow fever virus, are very difficult to grow outside of the host's body. They must be cultivated in special animal models or in cell cultures. At first, viruses were inoculated into chicken eggs to study their life cycle. However, this gave no evidence about the disease caused by the virus. Human cell cultures are now carried out in a way that shows the disease capability of the virus. The researchers can monitor the cellular responses to the virus the represent the course of the diseases in the human body.

Epidemiological research today is conducted in two ways. One way investigates the occurrence of a disease after it already happened. This method is called **retrospective epidemiology**.

Another way, called **prospective epidemiology**, determines whether a disease may happen in a person or a population in the future. Prospective epidemiology is more accurate when it is supported by retrospective epidemiological studies carried out over a period of years. The most common form of epidemiological investigation uses retrospective methods principally for new types of diseases. These studies help scientists collect comprehensive data about the factors that forecast the occurrence of a disease. A retrospective study on a new disease or a disease in an unexpected population of people is called a **case-control study**. Early case-control studies helped distinguish yellow fever from other types of fever diseases that were prevalent when yellow fever was discovered.

Epidemiologists require large amounts of detailed medical data to collect retrospective information. They gather this information from historical accounts of a disease and from current medical records. In many parts of the world, physicians are asked to report the occurrences of diseases to the Centers for Disease Control and Prevention or the World Health Organization. The Centers for Disease Control and Prevention is a federal organization in the United States that monitors diseases. Global diseases are studied by the World Health Organization, which is a branch of the United Nations that monitors diseases. The information for a particular disease is statistically analyzed to determine the common conditions and causes associated with the disease. This information in turn is used to predict situations in which the disease can occur.

Epidemiologists have many concepts that are important for understanding yellow fever. The term *risk factor* explains the circumstances that cause a person to develop a disease. A risk factor can be due to some attribute of the person, making him or her more susceptible to a disease. Certain genetic conditions related to the body's ability to fight disease are one type of risk factor. Personal habits such as the quality of a person's diet and the amount of stress in his or her life are examples of behavioral risk factors.

Exposure is an environmental risk factor that increases the chance of acquiring a disease. The environmental risk factors for yellow fever are any situation that brings the virus in contact with the person. The time between the measurable onset of disease and detection of the diseases is called the **latent period. Morbidity** is used to describe any illness resulting from a disease. **Mortality** is a measure of the number of deaths from a disease in a particular population of people during a particular period of time.

Another important term describes the way a disease is transmitted through a population. **Carrier** refers to a person or animal that shows no evidence of the disease but carries the infectious agent. A carrier can unknowingly spread disease to other people. People who have a mild and undetectable form of yellow fever can pass the disease to mosquitoes. **Contagious** is the term that describes the ease with which a disease can be transmitted from one person to another. **Endemic** describes the regular presence of a disease or infectious agent in a certain group of people. The term **epidemic** is used to explain the occurrence of more cases of disease than expected in a given area or among a specific group of people within a certain period of time. A **pandemic** describes the global occurrence of a disease. Any sudden, violent, spontaneous occurrence of a disease is called an **outbreak**.

EPIDEMIOLOGY OF YELLOW FEVER

The epidemiology of yellow fever was at first very difficult to understand. Nobody knew where the disease originated and little was known about its cause or transmission. Although yellow fever originated in Africa, the first reliable account of yellow fever was recorded in the Yucatan peninsula in 1648. An earlier account of what was thought to be yellow fever appeared in Barbados in 1647. The disease in Barbados was called *coup de barre* (fatigue) and could likely have been yellow fever. However, it was not confirmed whether the disease was yellow fever. At first, it was thought that the disease was native to the

Americas because of this first appearance in Mexico. There is speculation that Christopher Columbus and his troops may have contracted yellow fever in 1492 during the battle of Vega Real in Hispaniola. However, they may have suffered from one of many conditions that resembled yellow fever.

Yellow fever was then identified in Africa in 1878 when large occurrences of the disease were killing many people in Senegal, including pharmacists and physicians. Public health officials at the time hypothesized that yellow fever likely started in Africa because it seemed to afflict Europeans and South American indigenous people more than Africans. They believed that over time Africans developed resistance against the disease. It was later learned that the yellow fever first discovered in the Americas was the same disease described by western Africans centuries earlier. Knowing the true origin of the disease did little for understanding how it was transmitted. However, scientists were aware that the incidence of yellow fever was related to warm, wet climates.

In the early 1800s, it was thought that either the bad air associated with standing water or the odors associated with rotting vegetation caused yellow fever. Both conditions were typical in places where yellow fever was prevalent. This hypothesis was also used to explain the spread of malaria, which had a similar epidemiology. Most physicians were not satisfied with this explanation and looked for other ways that these environmental conditions could cause disease. Then, in 1848, American physician Josiah Nott hypothesized that mosquitoes likely spread certain diseases, including yellow fever, to humans. In 1881, Cuban physician Carlos Finlay proposed that the *Aedes aegypti* mosquito was the likely yellow fever vector. His work was confirmed by Walter Reed and his research team in 1901. This finding established that yellow fever originated in Africa where *Aedes aegypti* naturally resides.

A virus was hypothesized as the probable cause of yellow fever years before it was isolated in 1927. Early attempts to

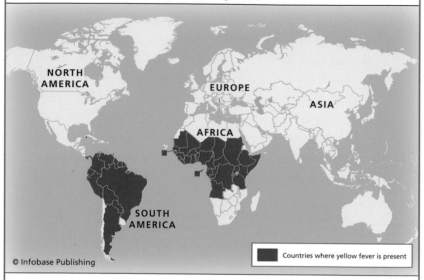

Approximate Global Distribution of Yellow Fever, by Country, 2007

NORTH AMERICA

EUROPE

ASIA

AFRICA

SOUTH AMERICA

© Infobase Publishing

■ Countries where yellow fever is present

Countries where Yellow Fever Is Present

Angola	Equatorial Guinea	Panama
Argentina	Ethiopia	Paraguay
Benin	French Guiana	Peru
Bolivia	The Gambia	Rwanda
Brazil	Gabon	São Tomé and Príncipe
Burkina Faso	Ghana	Senegal
Burundi	Guinea	Sierra Leone
Cameroon	Guinea-Bissau	Somalia
Central African Republic	Guyana	Sudan
Chad	Kenya	Suriname
Congo	Liberia	Tanzania
Congo, DRC	Mali	Trinidad and Tobago
Colombia	Mauritania	Togo
Côte d'Ivoire (Ivory Coast)	Niger	Uganda
Ecuador	Nigeria	Venezuela

Figure 3.3 The current distribution of regular yellow fever outbreaks is in Africa and South America. Yellow fever is currently a primary concern in countries that have little funds for health care and have few resources to perform adequate epidemiological research.

isolate the causative agent of yellow fever showed that it was an unfilterable agent. The yellow fever virus was discovered concurrently by British scientist Adrian Stokes in Nigeria and by French researchers Constant Mathis and Jean Laigret at the Dakar Pasteur Institute in Senegal. Both teams used monkeys as a model to isolate the virus. This final unraveling of the yellow fever "mystery" helped scientists fully explain the spread of the disease and to carry out effective prospective epidemiology studies that could be used to prevent the spread of yellow fever.

Yellow fever remains endemic in Africa. The slave trade introduced the disease to the Caribbean, Central America, South America, and the United States. It remains in South America where it is now an endemic disease. Small outbreaks occur globally. This is temporary and due to the unintentional importation of infected mosquitoes, particularly into Asia. A 1998 World Health Organization report estimates that each year yellow fever infects 200,000 people worldwide and results in approximately 30,000 deaths. The major carrier for the disease is infected humans. However, monkeys also carry the disease. Yellow fever is then spread to humans who live in proximity to the infected monkeys and biting insects. The disease is contagious in areas high in biting insect populations.

The number of cases of yellow fever in Africa and Latin America has fluctuated greatly since people began monitoring the disease carefully in 1906. Much of this was due to human migrations from rural to urban areas. Researchers discovered that rural people who had not been exposed to the disease acquired infections that were endemic to large urban areas. Their immune systems were not prepared to fight off the virus. Yellow fever occurred very infrequently in Africa and Latin America between 1980 and 1985 as a result of mosquito control and vaccination programs. The incidence of yellow fever then significantly rose in Africa, reaching epidemic proportions by 1988. Most of the cases occurred in unvaccinated children whose families had little access to medical care. After a dramatic decrease of the disease in 1989, occurrences of yellow fever again rise and fall, primarily in Africa. Its appearance remains infrequent and sporadic in Latin America.

The mortality rates from yellow fever vary greatly from one country to another. In the Ivory Coast, yellow fever resulted in

Table 3.1 Yellow fever epidemiological data for Africa, 2004

Country	Number of cases	Number of deaths	Case-fatality rate (%)
Ivory Coast	92	4	4%
Burkina Faso	14	6	43%
Guinea	6	0	0%
Cameroon	6	0	0%
Liberia	5	5	100%
Senegal	2	0	0%
Mali	2	1	50%
Ghana	1	0	0%

Source: World Health Organization, 2005.

four deaths in 2004, whereas in Liberia all five infected people died (Table 3.1). The death rate is more consistent in South America, averaging about 50 percent (Table 3.2).

Two major risk factors for yellow fever mortality are access to health care and diet. A lack of health care prevents people from seeking medical **treatments** that reduce the body damage caused by the virus. **Malnutrition** and undernutrition, usually resulting from poverty, weaken the body's immune defenses and make it more likely for the virus to harm major body organs. Children are the group that is most likely to die as a result of the disease, because the virus is capable of damaging a greater proportion of the body than in adults. War and forced migrations contribute to the diminished health care and increase in poverty.

The globalization of yellow fever began with the slave trade and is now a consequence of the technologies associated with modern society. Today, international commerce, world travel, and modern warfare contribute greatly to the spread of the

Table 3.2 Yellow fever epidemiological data for South America, 2004

Country	Number of cases	Number of deaths	Case-fatality rate (%)
Peru	61	31	51%
Colombia	30	11	37%
Bolivia	10	4	40%
Brazil	5	3	60%
Venezuela	5	3	60%

Source: World Health Organization, 2005.

insect vectors and the distribution of infected individuals. The disease remains restricted to climates and conditions that keep the virus alive in appropriate hosts and maintain a year-round, permanent population of the vectors. This is also true for other diseases such as malaria and sleeping sickness. Both of these diseases share a similar history to yellow fever.

4

Diagnosis, Treatment, and Prevention

Confirming the diagnosis of an infectious disease can be very frustrating when the organism causing the disease cannot be isolated from the body. In 1972, during a prolonged yellow fever outbreak, nine adult male patients from the Jos Plateau of Nigeria were admitted to the hospital with conditions resembling yellow fever. They had headaches, high fever, muscle pain, nausea, and they were vomiting blood. Several of the patients reported having these signs and symptoms for as long as two months. Although these conditions are typical of yellow fever, they could have been caused by a variety of diseases found in northwestern Africa. A series of blood tests, tissues sample analyses, and urine tests were conducted on the patients to identify whether the conditions were due to yellow fever.

All the patients showed enlargement of the liver, which could have been caused by other viral diseases, including hepatitis. Proteins found in the urine of these patients indicated some type of kidney damage. Again, this could have been due to a condition other than yellow fever. Test after test showed body conditions that can indicate other infectious disorders. Ten days of blood and liver tests gave conflicting results. Earlier testing appeared to indicate yellow fever, but later testing led the physicians to believe that other viral diseases were present. Unfortunately, no viruses were found in any of the patient's bodies. Sensitive tests for detecting viruses did not exist in the 1970s, and these cases were never confirmed to be yellow fever. This made it difficult to track the spread of the outbreak. Yellow fever is often confused with dengue fever, hemorrhagic fever, leptospirosis, malaria, and viral hepatitis during diagnosis.[1]

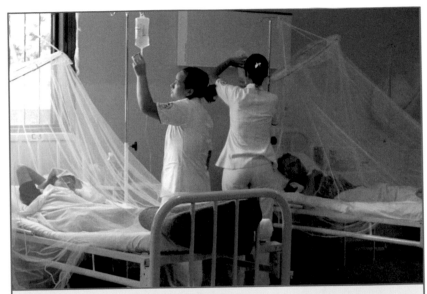

Figure 4.1 Patients suffering from yellow fever at a hospital in Asuncion, Paraguay, in February 2008. (© Cristaldo/epa/Corbis)

DIAGNOSIS OF YELLOW FEVER

The ability of a physician to identify a particular disease requires a process called the **diagnosis**. Physicians typically make a **presumptive diagnosis** of a disease by doing a physical examination. During the physical examination the physician collects visual indicators of disease **signs**. Signs are visible or measurable characteristics of a disease. The physician also records information about **symptoms** reported by the patient. Symptoms are subjective features such as headache or feeling chilled. From this information, the physician then narrows the presumptive diagnosis to likely disease condition. Making a presumptive diagnosis for yellow fever is very difficult because it resembles many other types of infectious disease.

Today most physicians supplement the presumptive diagnosis examination with standard medical history forms. The form is used to collect information about a patient's current general health and past conditions that could affect the diagnosis, **prognosis**, and treatment of a disease. Previously taken medications and prior medical treatments are also reported on this form. A separate physical examination form is then filled out by the physician to record major observable signs and symptoms. The physician then submits a form requesting clinical tests from a medical laboratory. This form is returned with laboratory information to help with the diagnosis of a suspected disease.

After the presumptive diagnosis, the physician orders **clinical tests** that give further information about the disease. Clinical tests include a large variety of medical testing done on body samples. These tests help determine the cause of a disease. Blood and urine are the two most commonly collected body fluids used for clinic testing. Occasionally, samples of cells and **mucus** are collected from the mouth and throat. This is commonly done to isolate microorganisms when an infectious disease such as yellow fever is suspected.

Diseases are generally diagnosed using standard diagnostic guidelines established by medical and governmental organizations. The **Clinical Surveillance Program** (CSP) is a program for diagnosing disease that was established by the National Institutes of Health. It bases a diagnosis on a growing database of accurately reported cases. The **Management Sciences for Health** (MSH) is a private, international nonprofit organization that works on public health issues that has developed its own system of diagnosis. The MSH definition provides a scientific explanation of the disease that facilitates consistent diagnosis. These definitions also serve as guidelines for the expected results for clinical tests that confirm the disease.

The CSP and MSH descriptions of yellow fever are generic descriptions of several flavivirus diseases, which helps public health practitioners recognize that other diseases caused by this virus have similar disease characteristics and may be confused for yellow fever. It also helps confirm that any clinical testing should be detecting flavivirus in the body if yellow fever is suspected. Yellow fever is described by MSH as:

> An acute infectious viral disease of short duration and varying severity. Typically, it is characterized by acute onset of fever, chills, headache, backache, generalized muscle pain, prostration, nausea, and vomiting. In addition, the pulse may be slow, weak, and out of proportion to the elevated temperature (i.e., Faget's sign). Most cases improve and recover within 3–4 days; however, about 15% enter into a second or toxic phase approximately 1 day of initial recovery. Symptoms of toxic phase include fever, jaundice, epistaxis, gingival bleeding, hematemesis (i.e., vomiting of blood, usually coffee-ground or black in color), Melina, and liver and renal failure. Twenty to 50% of jaundiced cases are fatal.

The definition warns that yellow fever must be differentiated from dengue fever, any hemorrhagic fever, leptospirosis, typhoid fever, and any viral hepatitis.

CSP and MSH also provide distinct definitions of flaviviruses to assist with the diagnosis of yellow fever. The CSP definition is more general and explains the flavivirus diseases in one statement:

> A family of RNA viruses, many of which cause disease in humans and domestic animals; there are three genera, Flavivirus, Pestivirus, and Hepacivirus, as well as several unassigned species.

The MSH definition of the yellow fever virus is:

> A genus of *Flaviviridae* containing several subgroups and many species. Most are arboviruses transmitted by mosquitoes or ticks. The type species is yellow fever virus.

Physicians use these definitions, along with the standardized diagnosis, to make the final diagnosis of yellow fever. In some cases, they must report confirmed cases of yellow fever to public health authorities.

The World Health Organization and public health agencies in many countries require physicians to complete a yellow fever surveillance document for each diagnosed case and purported outbreak of the disease. Many warm regions in the United States, such as Texas, require physicians to fill out a Mosquito Borne Illness Case Investigation Form used to report dengue fever, California encephalitis, eastern/Venezuelan/western equine encephalitis, St. Louis encephalitis, West Nile fever, and yellow fever. This information is needed to avert possible outbreaks.

SIGNS AND SYMPTOMS OF YELLOW FEVER

Yellow fever is a highly variable disease that presents different signs and symptoms depending on the patient's age, disease history, nutritional health, and general physical condition. Initial exposure to the bite with an infected mosquito or biting insect starts the **incubation period** of yellow fever. It usually takes three to six days for the yellow fever virus to replicate a large enough number of viral particles to produce disease. There are usually no signs or symptoms of the disease during the incubation period.

The incubation period leads to the infection or invasion stage. This lasts for two to five days after the end of the incubation period. The viruses are now reproducing rapidly and traveling throughout the body. Immune system chemicals called **pyrogens** cause the rapid onset of a fever that reaches 102 to 104°F (39 to 40°C). As the fever appears, the patient's heart rate speeds up and then slows down on the next day. This cycling of the heart rate (Faget's sign), which is usually determined by the pulse, continues for about three days. Faget's sign is a clinically important period because it indicates that the viruses can be detected in the patient's blood, so a blood sample is usually collected during this stage. It is very difficult for physicians to differentiate yellow fever from other infectious diseases at this point.

Physicians also request a **cerebrospinal fluid** test and an **electrocardiogram** (EKG) to help diagnose yellow fever. The cerebrospinal fluid is tested for evidence of bacteria, bacterial toxins, blood, immune system cells, and enzymes. Testing for bacteria helps determine the cause of the disease and also checks for other infections that result from a viral attack. The other measurements determine if an infection is taking place and assess any damage to the brain and spinal cord. An EKG is a medical procedure that measures the electrical activity of the heart. It provides detailed information about heart functions that are specifically produced by different types of diseases. Certain heart activities can be associated with yellow fever and related viral disorders.

Many people in yellow fever–prone areas show mild signs and symptoms as the infection stage progresses. They may have a flushed face, headaches, nausea, and redness of the eyes. These signs and symptoms can last one to three days. Other signs and symptoms appear in severe cases, including constipation, dizziness, irritability, muscle pains in the legs and along the back, restlessness, stomach distress, decreased urination, vomiting, and weakness. Children may exhibit **seizures**.

The most extreme cases of yellow fever produce black vomit and the breakage of blood vessels throughout the body (hemorrhaging). This is sometimes seen as bleeding from the gums and nose. The black color of the vomit is due to decayed blood. People with weakened immune systems due to other diseases or nutritional deficiencies become susceptible to other infections at this stage. Again, even these extreme conditions of yellow fever resemble several other viral diseases.

A **remission** stage follows the infection stage, usually five days after the end of the incubation period. The remission stage is indicated by a decrease in the disease signs and symptoms. It makes the patient believe that the body has fought off the disease and that he or she is getting better. This stage can last five hours to several days. Some people recover entirely from yellow fever at this stage. The immune system is aggressively fighting the disease at this point and may completely eliminate the virus from the body. Many people progress to the next part of the yellow fever sequence called the **intoxication** stage.

The intoxication stage is characterized by fever, jaundice (yellowing of the skin and eyes), and bleeding from the nose, rectum, and vagina. Vomiting begins again, as does the slowing of the heart rate (bradycardia) that was typical in the infection stage. The virus is now doing great damage throughout the body systems and kills cells of the kidneys, liver, and lungs. Organ failure can occur at this stage. Physicians also notice clinical test results that show high levels of proteins in the urine, dehydration, low blood sugar (hypoglycemia), and chemical evidence of kidney damage. Red dots (petechiae and ecchymoses) may appear on the skin, caused by damage to small blood vessels. The patient's feces are usually very dark (melena) and dry. These signs and symptoms can continue for three to nine days. The virus is very difficult to detect in the blood during this stage because most of the virus particles are replicating in the different organs.

About 50 percent of the patients never enter **convalescence** and die 10 to 14 days after the beginning of the intoxication stage. Physicians notice that fatal cases of yellow fever are preceded by convulsions, extreme disorientation, lowering of the body temperature (hypothermia), and severe hypoglycemia. Some patients go into a coma before dying. In less severe cases of yellow fever, convalescence follows the intoxication stage. Permanent organ damage can result, making the body susceptible to other illnesses.

CLINICAL TESTING OF YELLOW FEVER

Yellow fever can only be confirmed if a physician requests specific tests that prove positive for the flavivirus that causes yellow fever. These tests are also necessary to determine the particular type of yellow fever virus causing the disease. They also help identify where the virus was contracted, because each type of yellow fever virus comes from a specific region of Africa, the Caribbean, or Latin America.

Special laboratory tests are needed to confirm yellow fever. The World Health Organization recommends that every country at risk of yellow fever outbreaks have at least one national laboratory where yellow fever blood testing can be done. The organization even provides training programs to help medical staff and public health officials perform and understand the test results. These tests, called diagnostic tests, look for direct evidence of the virus in the body. Diagnostic tests can be done to measure the viral genome, viral attachment proteins called antigens, and immune system proteins called **antibodies**. Another test using a microscopic examination of infected body samples can be used to confirm yellow fever.

Viral genetic material is tested by collecting blood or tissue samples from the patient. The viral genome is found in very low concentrations in the body even in heavy infections, so a procedure called a **polymerase chain reaction** (PCR) is performed to make multiple copies of the viral RNA. A special modification of the PCR reaction called RNA amplification is performed because PCR was developed to multiply DNA. The RNA is then analyzed using a procedure called **electrophoresis**, by which molecules can be separated according to size and electrical charge as a means of identification. This technique is good for distinguishing between the different types of yellow fever viruses.

The other diagnostic testing uses **immunohistochemistry** to identify the virus or antibodies. Immunohistochemistry is a chemical procedure that uses antibodies to detect the presence of disease organisms. The most common tests use one system called enzyme-linked immunosorbent assay (ELISA) and another called microsphere-based immunoassay (MIA). Both techniques use antibodies glued to a substrate to isolate and detect particular types of proteins. The antibodies used in ELISA and MIA stick specifically to yellow fever attachment proteins and antibodies against the yellow fever virus. The tests look for the presence of an antibody called **immunoglobin G** (IgG).

Other types of tests called serological examinations use blood cells and immune system components called complements to detect viral proteins or antibodies. Both tests have methods of detecting whether the viral proteins or antibodies are sticking to the test chemicals. Histopathology requires putting a patient's tissue samples under a **microscope** and comparing them to healthy samples and specimens with yellow fever.

Clinical testing for yellow fever can take several days, meaning that the disease can progress and worsen before the results are confirmed.

TREATMENT OF YELLOW FEVER

There are no historical records of specific treatments for yellow fever preceding its identification in the 1600s. Yellow fever resembled a host of other diseases and was treated with traditional medicines and **therapies** that reflected the beliefs of the culture. It is likely that people were given herbal **remedies** or took part in spiritual rituals to rid the body of disease. From the 1600s through the late 1800s, physicians were at a loss when trying to treat yellow fever. No cures were available and treatment consisted primarily of bed rest, water, and food. Medications such as willow bark, which contains aspirin, and quinine were given to reduce the fever.

Dr. James Wilson, in a classic 1911 book called *Infectious Disease,* provided a detailed description of yellow fever treatments used from the late 1800s through the early 1900s. His writing reflects the frustration that physicians experienced while treating viral diseases. In the book he states:

> There is no known remedy which will abort or cure yellow fever. No drugs appear to possess the slightest influence upon the pathological process. Recovery occurs spontaneously in about 50 per cent, of the cases, no mat-

ter what form of treatment is adopted. Sanarelli's **serum** treatment has been almost entirely abandoned. Among the remedies which are most widely used in the treatment of yellow fever are quinine and sodium salicylate. Upon careful study, it has been shown that the salts of quinine are rather harmful than useful and have only shown beneficial effects in those cases in which malaria and yellow fever coexisted. Sodium salicylate has only been found efficacious in benign cases which would have recovered under any other form of treatment (Sodre and Couto).

The majority of physicians in tropical countries in which yellow fever is endemic advise an active expectant treatment. Upon the first day of the disease in all cases diaphoretics and laxatives are administered. Thus, in mild cases, a mustard foot bath and warm drinks or ammonium acetate are employed. If the case is more severe, if there is decided fever and marked pain, besides the mustard foot bath and local sinapisms, either of the following formulae are prescribed..." [2]

In the book he lists a variety of drugs and toxic substances that are no longer or rarely used in medicine. Included are various mixtures of silver filtrate, lead acetate, iron, Jamaican rum, antipyrini, tincture aconiti, syrup aurant, sulfur, ergot, julep gummos, xatrii salicylate, opium, cocaine, calomel, caster oil, and rhubarb juice. He suggested giving these drug treatments during the infection stage of the disease until the patient begins to sweat profusely. The patient is then induced to vomit with acidic drinks or certain plant oils such as castor oil. Iron was given to make up for blood loss if the patient was producing black vomit. Cocaine and opium were legal drugs then and were used to reduce the painful symptoms. Wilson also recommended cold sponge baths and ice packs on the head to control the fever and reduce headaches. The intoxication stage of yellow fever was treated with hot baths and opium. The mixture of drugs used in the infectious stage was given again during the convalescence stage until all signs and symptoms of the disease were gone.

Today, there are no **antiviral** drugs for treating yellow fever. Physicians normally administer what is called supportive care. Supportive care involves any strategy that makes the patient comfortable and reduces any body damage caused by the disease. For yellow fever, the typical supportive care includes giving plenty of water to make up for fluids lost during vomiting. Oxygen is also provided to make up for the gas exchange lost by the damaged lungs. Medications may be administered to regulate the blood pressure and the heart rate. Patients with severe yellow fever my need blood and **kidney dialysis**. Some patients need transfusions of blood liquids to replace proteins that improve blood clotting and healing of damage from hemorrhaging.

PREVENTION OF YELLOW FEVER

The first systematic plan for preventing yellow fever was applied immediately after Walter Reed discovered that mosquitoes transmitted the disease. The American government carried out mosquito control methods as a way of reducing the spread of yellow fever. This was accomplished by draining water from mosquito breeding grounds and adding oil to large bodies of water to kill off young mosquitoes. Government personnel and military troops working in areas with yellow fever were provided with mosquito netting to ward off bites in the field and when sleeping.

During World War II, pesticide spraying became a common means of controlling yellow fever in Asia where battles were taking place (Figure 4.2). Many of these sprays, such as DDT (dichloro-diphenyl-trichloroethane), were banned in the 1970s because they proved hazardous to human health and wildlife. Alternatives to DDT are not as effective in controlling mosquitoes. So, some countries keep using DDT despite the environmental and health concerns.

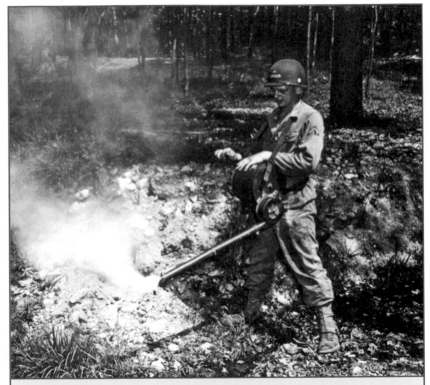

Figure 4.2 A soldier sprays pesticide to control mosquitoes carrying yellow fever, 1945. (National Library of Medicine)

Hospitals usually treat yellow fever patients in rooms that are kept free from mosquitoes. The patients may even be placed in beds covered with mosquito netting. This strategy reduces the chance of mosquitoes picking up the virus from infected patients. Public health officials in many warm areas regularly collect mosquitoes for yellow fever testing. The virus is detected using the same immunohistochemistry techniques performed on human specimens.

Today the Centers for Disease Control and Prevention recommend certain guidelines for yellow fever control, and the World Health Organization suggests similar precautions. The following guidelines are useful for reducing the incidence of any disease spread by mosquitoes and biting flies:

1. *Use insect repellent.* On exposed skin when you go outdoors, use an EPA-registered insect repellent such as those with DEET, picaridin, or oil of lemon eucalyptus. Even a short time outdoors can be long enough to get a mosquito bite.

2. *Wear proper clothing to reduce mosquito bites.* When weather permits, wear long sleeves, long pants, and socks when outdoors. Mosquitoes may bite through thin clothing, so spraying clothes with repellent containing permethrin or another EPA-registered repellent will give extra protection. Don't apply repellents containing permethrin directly to skin.

3. *Be aware of peak mosquito hours.* The peak biting times for many mosquito species is dusk to dawn, however *Aedes aegypti,* the main vector of yellow fever virus, feeds during the daytime. Take extra care to use repellent and protective clothing during daytime as well as evening and early morning or consider avoiding outdoor activities during these times when in areas where yellow fever is a risk.[3]

Air-conditioning has unexpectedly contributed to the decline of yellow fever. It reduces exposure to the mosquitoes because there is no need to cool houses by keeping windows and doors open.

Vaccination has become a very effective means of controlling yellow fever (Figure 4.3). The first yellow fever vaccine was developed by South African physician Max Theiler in 1927. He produced what is called a live **attenuated** vaccine prepared from 17D yellow fever virus strain raised in chicken eggs. Attenuated vaccines are made by weakening the virus with chemicals that either disable the attachment proteins or damage the RNA genome. The attenuated virus is able to produce an immune response but is unable to replicate in the host cells.

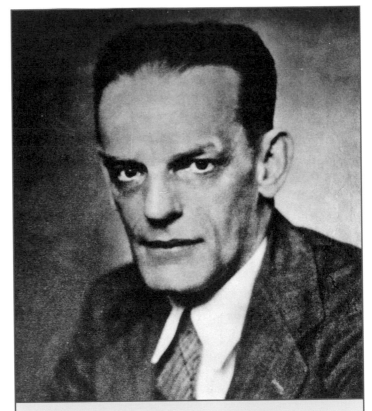

Figure 4.3 South African physician Max Theiler developed the first yellow fever vaccine in 1927. (National Library of Medicine)

Vaccines cause the body to produce a rapid immune response against the virus upon infection. This prevents the virus from reproducing immediately in the body after being infected. In unvaccinated people, the virus replicates faster than the body can attack it. This early yellow fever vaccine was first tested in New York in 1936 and in Brazil in 1937. Theiler was awarded the 1951 Nobel Prize for Physiology or Medicine for developing the vaccine. The modern version of the yellow fever vaccine is called YF-Vax and is administered as a needle injection. Physicians use the term **parenteral** when referring to injected drugs.

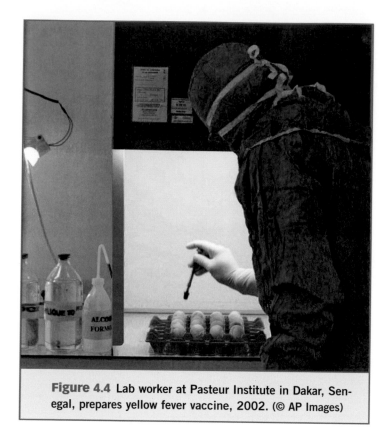

Figure 4.4 Lab worker at Pasteur Institute in Dakar, Senegal, prepares yellow fever vaccine, 2002. (© AP Images)

Vaccinating against yellow fever is suggested for residents in high-risk areas for people nine months of age and older. Travelers to Africa, Asia, South America, and certain Caribbean nations should also be vaccinated. The vaccine provides effective immunity for 10 years. The vaccine is not recommended for children six to nine months old or pregnant women. These individuals should be vaccinated only if an outbreak is present and they cannot be guarded from mosquito bites. Vaccinations are normally not given to infants under four months old because of possible health complications, but the vaccine does not affect the safety of breast milk and will not harm a breast-feeding infant.

Any side effects from the vaccine are mild and only occur in 25 percent of those vaccinated. Side effects may include headache, muscle aches (myalgia), and a slight fever a few days after vaccination. The vaccine's side effects typically last five to 10 days. Many people have painful swelling around the injection site. A mild, itchy rash covering large parts of the body develops in 1 percent of vaccinated people. People with egg **allergies** may show complications to the YF-Vax vaccine. The severity of side effects depends on the patient's sensitivity to the egg allergy.

Two rare adverse reactions are associated with yellow fever vaccine. One condition is called yellow fever vaccine– associated neurotropic disease, or postvaccinal **encephalitis,** and has occurred in only 10 patients since the use of the vaccine. It has a 50 percent fatality rate and causes damage to the brain and multiple body organs. The condition is more likely to occur in infants and in people with extremely weakened immune systems. Another condition is called

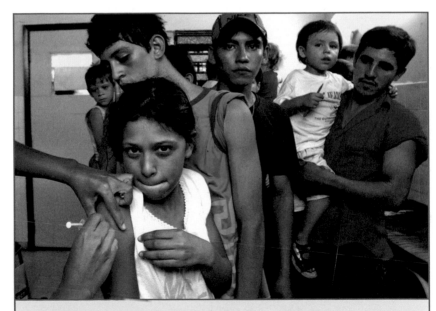

Figure 4.5 People line up for yellow fever vaccination in Paraguay. Yellow fever vaccination programs have dramatically reduced disease outbreaks. (© AP Images)

yellow fever vaccine–associated viscerotropic disease. It has only shown up in four people and causes fever associated with liver failure.

Global efforts to control yellow fever have reduced the disease but have not eliminated it. Outbreaks continue to occur and the disease sometimes appears in areas that do not have endemic yellow fever. Yellow fever continues to be a human plague and affects the livelihood of many people.

5

Yellow Fever and Other Modern Plagues

Philadelphia was the largest and most urbanized American city in 1798. Modern conveniences such as combination locks, fire extinguishers, flush toilets, self-winding clocks, and telegraphs could be found in many businesses and homes. Contemporary public practices and medicine kept down the spread of many of the infectious diseases found in less developed cities in the United States. However, this apparent protection from disease eroded in July 1798, when boatloads of refugees came to Philadelphia from the Caribbean. These people were leaving the territorial wars in the Caribbean as various European countries were battling for control of particular islands.

The refugees took many possessions with them. Unfortunately, many of the people unknowingly brought along items containing insects capable of spreading infectious diseases. These insects swarmed the docks of Philadelphia, creating a dangerous nuisance. One particularly dangerous pest was a type of mosquito that carries yellow fever. Yellow fever was prevalent in the Caribbean in the eighteenth century. More than 2,000 people became infected and died from a severe plague shortly after the invasion of the mosquitoes in Philadelphia in 1798. This plague caused many people to flee the city, including President George Washington and his staff. Philadelphia served as the nation's capital in 1798. The disease remained a mystery to physicians of the time. It is now known through examination of historical accounts and medical records that the disease was yellow fever.[1]

YELLOW FEVER AS A VIRAL PLAGUE

Yellow fever is one of many human diseases that had reached the status of being called a plague. The term *plague* is a middle French word for affliction, calamity, evil incident, or scourge. It has been in use since 1382. Plague was derived from the Latin word *plaga,* for "pestilence." The Latin language borrowed it from a similar Greek word *plaga,* which means "to hit." After 1601, many people used the term plague specifically for the disease black plague. Plague diseases typically had severe effects on the body, had a high fatality rate, and appeared as epidemics. Many early plagues were believed to be punishments imposed by God.

Viral plagues punished early people because of the mystery they posed and the devastation they produced. People were unaware of the causes of these plagues, and did not have the knowledge to treat and stop the spread of the diseases. Their perceptions of disease were influenced by misunderstanding and superstition. History has shown that yellow fever can be grouped with some of the most infamous viral plagues affecting humanity—Ebola, flu, HIV, and smallpox. These four diseases along with yellow fever were so feared that they immobilized cooperative global efforts to treat and eradicate the plagues.

EBOLA

Ebola, like yellow fever, is a viral hemorrhagic disease that seemingly appeared from nowhere and had a mysterious mode of transmission. Also like yellow fever, Ebola was ostensibly a new disease with the first confirmed cases appearing in the Democratic Republic of Congo (then known as Zaire) in 1976. This first outbreak infected 318 people and killed 280 of those people. There were periodic Ebola outbreaks in Gabon, Sudan, Uganda, and the Democratic Republic of Congo between 1976 through 2007. This pattern of Ebola outbreaks interestingly resembled the first occurrences of yellow fever in Africa, the Caribbean, and South America. Like yellow fever, it started

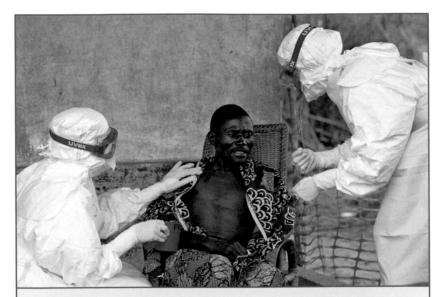

Figure 5.1 Congolese Ebola patient with workers from Doctors Without Borders. Public health officials need extra precautions when controlling Ebola. Mosquito protection is the major precaution when working in yellow fever areas. (© AP Images)

out as a disease of unknown origin that killed many people in sporadic outbreaks.

Ebola is caused by a filovirus belonging to the *Filoviridae* family. It has only one relative in the *Marburgvirus family*. There are five distinct varieties of Ebola virus: Côte d'Ivoire, Bundibugyo, Reston, Sudan, and Zaire. Like yellow fever, scientists believe that Ebola was originally a monkey disease that spread to humans. Filovirus diseases were discovered in 1967 in Marburg, Germany, when laboratory workers contracted an unknown disease from African green monkeys. The disease proved highly infectious, affecting 31 people. Seven of the people died from the virus. Unlike yellow fever, it was spread by direct contact with infected people. This made the disease more difficult to control than yellow fever.

Yellow fever made its way around the world as the consequence of the slave trade and international commerce. However, its persistence as a plague was restricted by the ability of the mosquito vector to survive and by the availability of wild monkeys to serve as an alternative host. Ebola is primarily limited to Africa. Outbreaks spread when people flee another outbreak, introducing the disease to a nearby country. The disease can spread rapidly throughout the population without the need of vectors or other hosts. It can remain indefinitely in an area once it is introduced, as long as infected people are present. Ebola accidentally made its way out of Africa in infected research monkeys exported to America, England, Italy, and the Philippines. One human case showed up in England. The English patient was a scientist who contracted the disease from a contaminated research sample.

Ebola is a more destructive disease than yellow fever. It causes severe internal bleeding. The disease appears four to six days after contact with the virus. It very rapidly produces a fever, sore throat, weakness, severe headache, joint pain, muscle aches, diarrhea, vomiting, dehydration, hacking cough, and stomach pain. The signs and symptoms are initially indistinguishable from yellow fever. External bleeding from body openings and sores occurs in extreme cases. There is no cure for Ebola and patients are given the same supportive treatments as yellow fever patients. Unlike yellow fever, there are currently no vaccines for Ebola. The only prevention strategy is to keep people away from infected individuals and outbreak areas.

FLU

Flu typically refers to a disease called influenza. However, it is also used to refer to other diseases of the respiratory system. The different flu diseases came about in epidemic proportions around the same time that yellow fever was making its way from Africa to the Americas and the Caribbean. The first use of the term *flu* was in Italy in 1357. It meant "to be under the influence," referring to being controlled by astrological influences of the stars. Yellow fever was also thought to have a spiritual cause and was perceived as a curse where it first appeared in Africa. Many people in the Americas and the Caribbean also viewed it as a scourge brought about by invisible fumes from stagnant water and filth.

Also like yellow fever, influenza and flu-like diseases produced sporadic outbreaks that made many people ill. It also had a similar mortality rate to yellow fever, making it an equally fearful plague. Unlike yellow fever, these diseases were spread by direct contact with the virus and did not require a living vector. They are more infectious than many other viral diseases because they are easily transmitted on nonliving objects called **fomites**.

The flu came to the Americas in 1580, before yellow fever was showing up in South America. It was brought to the Americas by European explorers and settlers. Several years later it became a pandemic disease affecting Asia, Africa, Europe and America. In total, over 90 percent of the world's population is vulnerable to flu outbreaks. Yellow fever has never truly reached pandemic status. Plus, it does not have the persistence of the flu diseases that generally remain endemic in the countries they affect.

Influenza, the "true flu," is caused by the influenza virus. It belongs to the orthomyxovirus family. Orthomyxoviruses affect a large variety of **vertebrate** animals. They are similar in structure to the flavivirus group to which yellow fever belongs. It is known that influenza started out as a pig disease that spread to humans during the development of animal agriculture. It is now known that animal **domestication** introduced many new diseases to humans.

Influenza is a highly variable disease ranging from very mild to highly fatal. At first, the signs and symptoms of influenza resemble yellow fever. The initial disease characteristics are fever, headache, muscle ache, tears, sensitivity of the eyes to light, dry cough, and a runny nose. Severe influenza can produce difficulty in breathing, lung damage, and bacterial lung infections. In rare cases the virus can damage the brain and heart. Unlike yellow fever, influenza does not cause bleeding and is typically localized in the respiratory system.

The flu-like diseases spread the same way as influenza and have many of the same signs and symptoms. These diseases can be caused by bacteria, fungi, protists, and viruses. Most flu-like diseases are caused by viruses. They are typically diagnosed as diseases with the following signs and symptoms: coughing up blood, rash, stiff neck, headache, sensitivity of the eyes to bright lights, drowsiness, confusion, vomiting, and chest pains. Avian flu, or **bird flu**, is the plague of this group primarily because of its pandemic status. Unlike yellow fever, avian flu viruses do not typically infect humans. It is a bird disease. The World Health Organization has an international surveillance program to detect and control any possible outbreaks.

Avian flu is caused by a variety of viruses related to influenza A. It belongs to a bird virus group called the H strains. This group is commonly found in domesticated birds such as chickens. It is believed that a type of the H strains developed a genetic **mutation** that permitted it to cause disease in humans. In humans, the disease is typically accompanied by cold viruses that exacerbate the signs and symptoms. Approximately 400 human cases have been reported since 2003. It is not known when the disease appeared and how many cases were confused with other diseases. Unfortunately, there are currently 15 H strains of bird flu viruses identified with illnesses in humans. Public health agencies are hoping it will never affect as many people as yellow fever. There is no cure for bird flu, and vaccinations do not guarantee protection from every type.

HIV

HIV, or human immunodeficiency virus, produces a disease called acquired immunodeficiency syndrome (AIDS). Like the yellow fever virus, HIV is an enveloped virus containing an RNA genome. However, it is a more specific virus and almost exclusively targets human **white blood cells**. It can invade other body cells as long as they are transported by white blood cells called T-cells. Unlike yellow fever, it is primarily contracted by sexual activity or contact with contaminated blood and body fluids. Initially, HIV had a very high mortality rate, killing almost all people infected with the virus. It left few survivors, unlike yellow fever, and quickly achieved plague status.

Viruses related to HIV emerged from the same area of West Africa as yellow fever. It was also a monkey disease, commonly infecting chimpanzees. It is believed to have initially spread to humans through the consumption of monkey meat. HIV strains with certain mutations were able to replicate in human cells. Viruses similar to HIV cause diseases in a variety of mammals including cats, dogs, and horses. It is likely present but undetected in many wild animals. Most of these viruses cause **cancers** and blood diseases in these animals. Cancers associated with HIV in humans is likely due to other sexually transmitted viruses that cause cancer.

Humans can be infected with two types of AIDS-associated HIVs: HIV 1 and HIV 2. There are multiple categories of HIV 1, which is subdivided into groups M, N, and O. Group M is further separated into 10 distinct types. More than 90 percent of HIV-1 infections belong to Group M. Group O is limited to West Africa and group N is found in Cameroon. The different types are associated with different regional outbreaks, as is true with yellow fever. HIV 1 is more easily transmitted and produces AIDS more rapidly. It is more difficult for HIV 2 to spread from person to person. HIV 2 takes longer to get established in the body and produces the AIDS condition more slowly than HIV 1.

HIV appears simpler to prevent than yellow fever. It can be avoided by restricting sexual contact. Safe sex practices reduce, but do not eliminate, its transmission. Unfortunately, many people still contract HIV because it is difficult to enforce global efforts to control the disease. Educational programs are not fully effective at changing the attitudes of people about unprotected sex. People are more likely to follow the mosquito management guidelines of yellow fever control. Contemporary AIDS treatments slow the development of the disease. However, they do not cure it or reduce its transmission. Unlike yellow fever, there are no effective vaccines against HIV.

SMALLPOX

Smallpox, like many of these modern plagues, has an uncertain history. Like yellow fever, it was probably confused with other diseases and not accurately reported in the medical literature. Like yellow fever, it was believed to have originated in Africa thousands of years ago. It then spread to Asia and Europe as people traveled for commerce, war, and new places to settle. Smallpox was a much greater plague than yellow fever, killing hundreds of millions of people since its official identification in 1350.

Outbreaks of smallpox appeared sporadically, much like yellow fever. However, its spread could not be as well predicted because it could not be associated with a particular feature of the environment. People knew that warm, wet climates were conducive to the spread and persistence of yellow fever. Unlike yellow fever, smallpox outbreaks occurred with less intensity over time after afflicting a particular region. It was later learned that people developed a strong immunity against the virus. This was not true for yellow fever, which produces a weaker body defense with a second infection.

The smallpox virus, or variola virus, belongs to the *Poxviridae* family. Its specific category is *Orthopoxvirus* and is related to two rare human diseases—molluscum contagiousum and variola—and to pox-like diseases in animals. Smallpox is likely to have originated in animals and spread to humans with the domestication of cattle. Cattle carry a similar disease called cowpox. Like yellow fever, this disease originated in animals. Like yellow fever, the pox viruses have an envelope; however, their genome is different because it is composed of DNA.

There is currently no cure for smallpox, as is true for most viral diseases. Smallpox prevention is difficult because it is easily spread and outbreaks are nearly impossible to predict. Smallpox ravaged the human population for many years before an effective campaign for controlling the disease was implemented. Yellow fever was quickly acted upon and was controlled effectively with

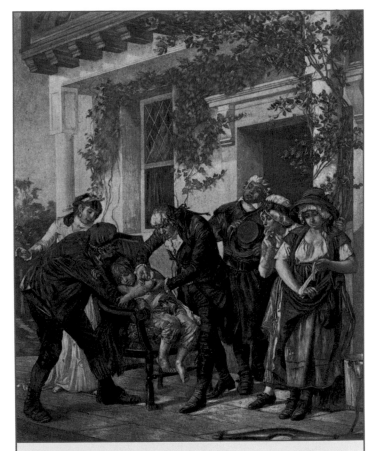

Figure 5.2 Edward Jenner inoculating a child against smallpox. Walter Reed's experiments on human subjects stirred as much debate as the testing of the first smallpox vaccine on humans by Edward Jenner in 1796. (Hierophant Collection)

the first vaccination and prevention programs in the early 1900s. A smallpox vaccine was developed in 1796 by English physician Edward Jenner However, its use was not widespread.

It was not until 1967 that the World Health Organization carried out a global initiative to eradicate smallpox. It took 10 years to accomplish the goal. This was achieved using a worldwide vaccination effort. A newer, more effective version of Jenner's vaccine was developed for the program. The last endemic case of smallpox appeared in 1977 in Somalia and no other cases occurred afterward. In 1980, the World Health Organization announced that the world was free of smallpox at the 33rd World Health Assembly meeting in Geneva, Switzerland.

YELLOW FEVER: AN EMERGING INFECTIOUS DISEASE

An emerging infectious disease is defined by the World Health Organization as an illness "that has appeared in a population for the first time, or that may have existed previously but is rapidly increasing in incidence or geographic range." Almost all of the great human plagues emerged from diseases that afflicted animals. These diseases resulted from mutations that gave the microorganisms the ability to invade human hosts. It is ironic that the conveniences brought about by modern society provided the environment for emerging diseases. These diseases are more likely to evolve in urban areas and in cultures that produced domesticated animals. They are also a consequence of modern global commerce and travel.

The World Health Organization and the public health organizations in many countries view emerging infectious diseases as a health care priority. They are hoping to prevent the reemergence of current diseases and hope to prevent outbreaks of any new infectious disease that may emerge. Emerging diseases have changed the course of human history. These diseases contributed to the outcomes of war, motivated immigration and emigration, changed cultural and religious practices, perpetuated prejudices, and encouraged creative ways of controlling disease. Emerging diseases have also caused people to rethink the way we live and altered the way people practice personal hygiene. These diseases have also made people more vigilant about the types of activities that promote disease.

6

The Impact of Diseases on History

A letter sent at midnight, December 31, 1900, by Walter Reed to his wife, Emilie, read, "Here I have been sitting reading that most wonderful book— La Roche on Yellow fever—written in 1853. Forty-seven years later it has been permitted to me & my assistants to lift the impenetrable veil that has surrounded the causation of this most dreadful pest of humanity and to put it on a rational & scientific basis."[1] The lifted "veil" discussed in the letter refers to Dr. Reed's lethal discovery of how yellow fever was contracted and spread. Yellow fever had cost millions of lives in sub-Saharan Africa and tropical South America since it was first recognized until the letter was written.

However, one person willingly gave his life to unveil how the disease was transmitted to people. Working in Water Reed's laboratory, the physician Jesse William Lazear deliberately exposed himself to mosquitoes thought to transmit yellow fever. He was an expert on diseases carried by mosquitoes. Without direct supervision from Reed, Lazear was testing the hypothesis that mosquitoes spread the yellow fever from one human to another. Lazear never claimed that he experimented on himself. However, Reed discovered self-experimentation evidence in Lazear's research notes after Lazear died from yellow fever on September 8, 1900. Lazear's death and severe illnesses incurred by other people from other yellow fever experiments on humans compelled the medical community to discourage deadly disease experiments on humans .[2]

IMPACT OF PLAGUES ON HUMANITY

Plagues significantly impacted the course of human history throughout recorded time. Archeological investigations on ancient human settlements even show that people were affected by plagues as far back as 40,000 years ago. Early plagues were viewed as punishments delivered from supernatural forces. Those afflicted by a plague were perceived either as wrongdoers or victims of unfortunate circumstances. Many of the early accounts of plagues were likely not accurate and were embellished to make the disease appear more insidious. Many religious writings, including the Bible, recorded plagues as factors that guided the moral and political decisions of the society.

International and civil wars were fought because of the black plague and related outbreaks. Poor people fought for lands that were once occupied by the rich landowners who succumbed to plague. Refugees escaping areas affected by the plague were met with violent resistance as they crossed into other municipalities. Countries sent armies to their borders to keep out immigrants who might be carrying the plague. Indigenous and nomadic tribes took full advantage of the plague-ravaged cities. They pillaged the weakened towns and attempted to settle these areas as new territories.

Plagues also had economic impacts on society because of the loss of many people in the workforce and the health care expenditures associated with recovering from large outbreaks. One modern example of the cost of plague was reported in a United Kingdom news story about a 1994 black plague outbreak in India. The article, entitled "Economic cost in excess of pounds 260m," stated that India's economy suffered primarily due to bans on business travel, tourism, international trade, monetary exchanges, and manufacturing. In addition, many people were too ill to work and purchase merchandise. The increase in medical care costs was only one small part of the economic decline from the disease. This great loss was incurred by an outbreak that was very small compared to the epidemics of earlier times. Approximately 1,700 suspected cases were reported. Only 693 cases were confirmed, with 50 deaths resulting from the outbreak. And yet an incredible loss of national revenue resulted from the brief outbreak, which lasted from August 26 through October 18, 1994.

The disease that probably had the greatest overall impact on human history was the black plague, which was also known as bubonic plague. It was a bacterial disease that became the modern symbol of all plagues that followed it. The disease was estimated to have killed 200 million people since it first hit the susceptible populations of Europe in about 1347. It is believed that the black plague outbreaks had taken place in the Mediterranean region between 450 B.C. and A.D. 540. Many epidemic outbreaks of black plague spread throughout Asia, Europe, and the Middle East until 1920. The scourge of black plague was reduced to small periodic outbreaks around the 1950s with the arrival of **antibiotics** and the implementation of rat and flea control programs.

Black plague, like yellow fever, was spread by biting insects. However, the vector was a flea and was not as noticeable as mosquitoes. The other host was a rat. Rats were found in high populations in European cities. The rats kept a fresh supply of the bacterium, *Yesinia pestis,* available for the fleas to spread to humans. This made the transmission of black plague a greater mystery than plagues like yellow fever. People were less likely to associate with one particular public health cause. Black plague perpetuated the belief that diseases were brought about by supernatural forces.

Other plagues, such as yellow fever, frightened societies because people did not ever want a repeat of the devastation brought about by black plague. Yellow fever was repeatedly referenced to black plague at the times of major yellow fever outbreaks. However, the black plague had some positive effect on how subsequent plagues were controlled. The public's confidence in religion and supernatural causes of disease decreased after the final onslaughts of the black plague. Much of this was due to the death of many clergy and pious people. Their faith

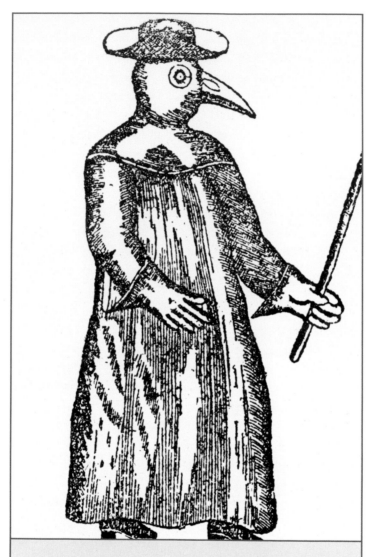

Figure 6.1 Black death suit used by doctors during Middle Ages as a preventive measure when visiting sick patients. The devastation brought about by black plague provided the incentive for society to take a more scientific approach to the investigation and control of subsequent plagues such as yellow fever.
(© Emilio Ereza/Alamy)

did not protect them from the disease. Many other people learned that prayer failed to prevent the plague from spreading its illness and death. Consequently, people became more and more reliant on scientifically valid methods to effectively control disease.

IMPACT OF YELLOW FEVER ON HUMANITY

The horrific outcomes of the black plague and other devastating human diseases paved the way for a rapid resolution to the yellow fever plague. Yellow fever was not discovered until much of the superstition about disease faded. However, the science of epidemiology was still in its infancy and was partly hindered by latent misconceptions about diseases. A misunderstanding of malaria led early researchers to believe the same incorrect information about the cause of yellow fever. It was fortunate that the strong desire to prevent yellow fever from reaching epidemic proportions inspired medical researchers to experiment on reasonable hypotheses about the disease.

In 1882, German **microbiologist** Robert Koch applied a new set of scientific principles in his efforts to discover the cause of the ancient plague **tuberculosis**. Tuberculosis, like a related disease called **leprosy**, was a well-documented disease in biblical times. It was at first associated with poverty, filth, and sin. In modern times, scientists took great efforts to find the actual cause of the disease with little success. Robert Koch developed an experimental strategy to confirm the identity of organisms causing infectious diseases. His method was later named "Koch's postulates." His postulates became the modern standard practice of infectious disease identification.

Koch's postulates required that an organism had to be isolated from a host suffering from the disease. The organism then had to be cultured in the laboratory for identification and characterization. This cultured organism then had to be introduced into another host to see if it caused the same disease. The organism then had to be re-isolated from that host and confirmed for the original identity. If carried out properly, Koch's method provided experimental evidence that a particular microbe traveling from host to host caused a specific condition. Koch's procedure helped Walter Reed's research team devise their strategy for coming up with the cause of yellow fever.

Reed concluded that an experimental method was the only way to quickly resolve the cause and spread of yellow fever. Unfortunately, Koch's postulates did not work for confirming the cause of yellow fever. The organisms could not be isolated and grown in culture for infection in another host. Plus, Koch was lucky to have animal models to investigate the diseases he worked with. Reed was unaware that yellow fever infected monkeys, so he thought that it would have to be studied on humans. The United States needed a quick end to yellow fever. The disease was causing chaos in every American city it affected. There were serious concerns that the upheavals caused by the black plagues would be repeated in the United States if yellow fever was not contained.

Reed's team first investigated the unsuccessful ideas behind yellow fever. The closest scientific hypothesis was proposed by the U.S. Army Surgeon General, George M. Sternbergin. He believed that an unknown bacterium was the cause of yellow fever. Sternbergin also thought that proper hygiene was the way to prevent its spread. Reed was appointed by Sternbergin with the mission of "pursuing scientific investigations with reference to the infectious diseases prevalent on the Island of Cuba." Initial investigations found no organism that could be cultured in a laboratory in yellow fever patients. This made it impossible to fulfill the requirements of Koch's postulates.

Reed was then compelled to perform experiments on living human subjects in his haste to find the cause of yellow fever. Careful human experimentation first indicated that mosquitoes passed the "invisible" agent one person to another. He then conducted other studies that established the timeline and course of the disease. Reed's team accomplished this by injecting the blood of yellow fever victims into healthy people. These investigations paved the way for the discovery of the yellow fever virus and its isolation from mosquitoes. Isolation of the virus then led to the development of the yellow fever vaccine. With all this information, the United States was able to carry out comprehensive yellow fever control efforts that dramatically reduced the incidence of yellow fever.

The heroic efforts of Reed's team created a medical ethics dilemma that changed human research forever. Accounts of the research caused consternation in the medical community. It was felt that Reed's team developed a dangerous precedent for medical research on human subjects. The research methods of his team went contrary to the Hippocratic Oath—that physicians are sworn to prevent any intentional harm to humans. Plus, it created public concern about the consent of human subjects taking part in medical experiments. Certain scientists found the yellow fever research unethical. They felt that it was "criminal" to intentionally inject a healthy human subject with a potentially lethal disease. Reed was forced to justify his research, claiming that he had full written consent from all of the research subjects. He was scrutinized in the same way Edward Jenner had been when he was criticized for testing the smallpox vaccine on humans in 1796.

The Nazi experiments on World War II prisoners of war and concentration camp prisoners solidified efforts to formulate international human research standards that protected the full rights of research subjects. The informed consent obtained by Reed was not nearly as detailed as the consenting documentation used today. In addition, studies have to be carefully reviewed by expert boards that evaluate the safety and rationale of the experimentation. These boards can also recommend alternative research that does not involve human subjects. Reed's yellow fever research unknowingly shaped landmark policies that protected the public from any prescription medication that could cause harm. His work also helped with the creation of safety regulations used in the production of food and household products.

PLAGUES AND WARFARE

The pursuit of a yellow fever cure was primarily driven by the need to protect troops from the disease during the Spanish-American War. Yellow fever, like other plague-causing organisms, regularly killed as many troops during wars as did the battles themselves. However, the cure was also important in another conflict. People wanted to combat the natural geology of the earth by building a shipping channel that would eliminate the need for cargo ships to circle South America as the only route from the East Coast to the West Coast of America. Unfortunately, the canal had to be excavated through Panama where yellow fever was rampant. Panama had the perfect climate and wet breeding grounds for flies and mosquitoes that carried yellow fever. The disease killed so many workers that it was impeding the progress of the construction, started by the French in 1880. Ultimately, the canal was completed by the United States in 1914 as the spread of yellow fever was being controlled.

Plagues also played a major role in how warfare was conducted. An early knowledge of plague led people to devise combat strategies using plague-infested materials as biological weapons. The first accurately documented account of biological warfare took place in 1346 during the siege of Kaffa in the Ukraine. Tartar soldiers catapulted the bodies of black plague victims into the city of Kaffa as a way of subduing their enemy. It was planned that the disease would spread among the city, making the residents too ill to fight. A plague did ensue, but it was more likely due to infected rats traveling from the Tartar campsites into the city of Kaffa. This strategy was used again in 1710 by the Russian army against the Swedish army during a battle in Estonia.

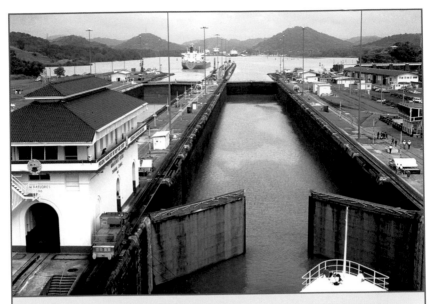

Figure 6.2 The building of the Panama Canal from 1880 though 1914 was hindered by many factors, including yellow fever. The climate and swampy terrain was a perfect breeding ground for the disease. (Dr. Edwin P. Ewing, Jr./CDC)

The first recorded use of biological warfare in North America involved smallpox as the weapon in 1767 during the French and Indian Wars. British troops at Fort Pitt in Pittsburg, Pennsylvania, took advantage of a smallpox outbreak that left many contaminated blankets in the medical hospital. The military planned to donate the blankets to local Indian tribes as a means of reducing the Native American population. A special ceremony was conducted and the Native Americans unknowingly accepted the infected blankets. The campaign proved successful because Native American tribes in the Ohio Valley succumbed to a smallpox epidemic after receiving the blankets.

Modern warfare made use of more sophisticated biological warfare methods. During World War I, the Germans tested the effectiveness of a bacterial disease called **anthrax** as a warfare agent. Cultures of bacteria were shipped to different war fronts in an attempt to kill off sheep, a major food source, and horses, a primary means of military transport. Fortunately for the American and Russian forces, the proposed project was never implemented. The fear of the dangers of this type of nontraditional warfare led to the 1925 Geneva Protocol for the Prohibition of the Use of Asphyxiating, Poisonous or Other Gases, and of Bacteriological Methods of Warfare. The treaty still exists and has been signed by many nations.

World War II provided the incentive to ignore the treaty. The United States and Japan started testing biological warfare agents. Japan killed thousands of Chinese people, testing a variety of biological warfare agents on citizens and prisoners. Major Chinese cities were assaulted with anthrax, cholera, salmonella and other biological agents. Many Japanese soldiers accidentally died in the attacks while handling the warfare agents. The Americans focused on anthrax as a weapon in warfare programs that were never implemented.

The favored organisms for biological warfare are microorganisms that spread easily from one host to another. Most of the organisms proposed for warfare selectively make humans ill. Some are targeted at economically important animals or plants as a means of disrupting or poisoning the food supply. Studies on yellow fever show that it is a feasible biological agent that can be distributed through contaminated mosquitoes. It can be used to cause temporary outbreaks that debilitate the population of a region. There is evidence that the yellow fever virus was developed into weapons by North Korea. In the 1960s, the United States performed yellow fever warfare studies in a program that has now been discontinued.

Plagues have brought about human suffering throughout the ages as natural diseases and as weapons of warfare. The devastation caused by plagues compelled people to create novel ways of rapidly combating their onslaught. These strategies have focused on disease cures, eradication, and prevention.

However, the microorganisms that cause plagues are constantly evolving, and over time they defeat people's best efforts to control them. Many countries are investigating high-tech methods of combating disease using strategies that will hopefully have lasting effects on the detection, prevention, and control of existing and emerging plagues.

7

Future Directions in Controlling Viral Diseases

Viruses are unlike other infectious microorganisms in that they do not possess the metabolic processes that carry out major life cycle functions. They rely completely on the resources of the host to replicate and find another host. The simplicity of viruses makes them very complicated to control when they are infecting a host cell. Most treatments have to harm the host in order to interfere with the viral life cycle. In addition, they are very difficult to destroy because their minimal structure resists many of the conditions that normally harm other organisms.

The cells of other microorganisms are easily disrupted by changes to their molecular structure. Because many of the drugs that kill other organisms would not work on viruses, it is difficult to disable them with common **disinfectants**. It is also difficult to disable a virus's life cycle, which requires interfering with the host cell metabolism and possibly killing the host cell. In other words, any drug that harms the virus would endanger the host. The spread of yellow fever is particularly problematic because scientists need to decide if it is best to control the disease in the mosquito or in the human host.

One way of dealing with viral diseases is by controlling their ability to replicate in host cells. This can be accomplished either by preventing viral binding to the host cells or by prohibiting the virus from replicating in the host cells. **Immunization** is the classic way of preventing viruses from entering host cells. One method of immunization involves the injection of

immunoglobulins into the bloodstream. Usually, large amounts are used and the injection is placed into a large area of muscle. Immunoglobulins stick to a variety of viruses, impeding their ability to attach to host cells.

Yellow fever is prevented by using another type of immunization called vaccination. Vaccination uses disabled viruses or part of the virus as an agent for stimulating the immune system to produce specific types of antibodies. The antibodies then attach to the virus, preventing it from attaching to host cells. Immune system chemicals then detect these virus particles and aid with the removal of the virus from the body. Vaccination also causes the body to develop a "memory" of the virus. This "memory" permits the body to fight off the virus very rapidly when another infection occurs. Vaccination is the preferred traditional way of controlling viruses. Traditional vaccines were made with viruses that were weakened by chemical treatments or by a special method of cultivating the virus. This method is very effective but can cause a mild illness that sometimes resembles the disease condition. In addition, certain vaccine viruses are raised in eggs and cause immune system problems for people with egg allergies. Vaccinations have an optimal lasting effect in the body for five years.

Medical researchers are using **biotechnology** to produce safer and longer-lasting vaccines. Scientists have learned that vaccines produce fewer side effects when only certain components of the virus are injected into the body. One type of vaccine is made from viral proteins that stimulate the greatest immune response in the body. Researchers have already identified attachment proteins in the yellow fever virus that cause the body to mount a rapid immune response. These attachment proteins can then be manufactured in a **genetically modified** bacterium containing a **gene** for that protein. The proteins are purified from the bacteria and turned into a vaccine that can be injected into the blood. No eggs are needed to raise the virus, which reduces the chance of a vaccine allergy.

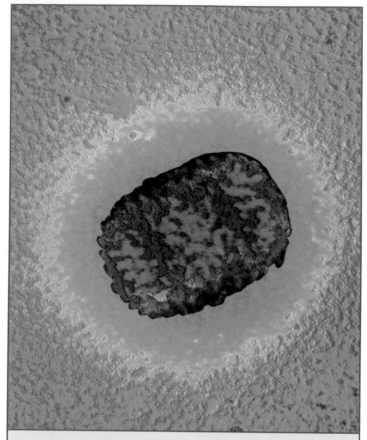

Figure 7.1 Electron micrograph of vaccinia virus. An artificial vaccinia virus may be the basis of a lifelong vaccine against viral diseases such as yellow fever. (© Institut Pasteur/Phototake)

Living artificial vaccines have also been investigated and may one day be used for yellow fever. Artificial viruses such as one called the vaccinia virus can be manufactured using biotechnology methods. This artificial virus can be programmed to live in the body without causing disease. Such viruses can be constructed to carry attachment proteins from the yellow fever virus. The artificial virus is then introduced into the body where it can replicate slowly as it induces a lifelong immunity against yellow fever without having any of the side effects of yellow fever vaccine. Research trials caused much concern that the vaccinia virus can cause a mild disease of its own. So, new investigations are focusing on using a vaccinia that cannot replicate. In effect, it acts as a safer form of the original yellow fever vaccine made from disabled yellow fever viruses. This form of vaccinia does not induce lifelong immunity.

Antiviral drugs are medications that alter the cell's metabolism in a way that impedes viral replication. One group of drugs uses this mechanism to prevent the viral genome from replicating. Another group interferes with capsid, or envelope, formation. This prevents the viruses from maturing. It can also work by preventing incomplete viruses from exiting the cell. In this way, the incomplete viruses become incapable of infecting other cells. Unfortunately, most antiviral drugs can harm the body. They can damage the blood-forming cells, kidneys, and liver. Certain antiviral drugs interfere with nerve cell function. Currently, antiviral drugs are most effective against the hepatitis virus, **herpes** virus, and the human immunodeficiency virus. There is no medication effective against the yellow fever virus.

Other medications are often given to supplement antiviral drugs. Immune system chemicals such as **interleukins** are given to boost the immune system's ability to remove viruses. An interleukin called **interferon** is regularly used to treat yellow fever. Alternative antiviral treatments are sometimes recommended to enhance traditional treatments. Many types of plant chemicals have mild antiviral activities. They are most effective in enhancing the body's ability to ward off a viral invasion. Most alternative treatments boost the immune system. They help the body remove viruses that have not yet entered cells or have recently exited an infected cell. Other alternative treatments interfere with a virus's ability to adhere to cells, thus limiting the replication rate of the viruses. In addition, these treatments help the mucous membranes remove viruses before the viruses have a chance of entering the cells.

One new therapy is being developed that specifically blocks capsid formation. It is called **interference RNA** therapy. The treatment involves an injection that introduces a molecule called interference RNA into the host's cells. Interference RNA then binds to the viral RNA blocking the virus's ability to manufacture capsids. This therapy may be a bonus for treating the yellow fever virus. Interference RNA may block replication of the viral RNA genome.

CONTROLLING VIRAL DISSEMINATION

Viral diseases are most successfully controlled at present with **prophylactic** strategies. The term prophylaxis means to avoid or stop something from occurring. Viral diseases are best thwarted by keeping the virus from contacting the cells of susceptible people. Methods for preventing viruses from entering the body vary greatly, depending on the viral life cycle. Cleanliness and personal hygiene are the simplest ways of keeping viruses from entering the body. Proper cleanliness removes viral particles attached to dust and to the surfaces of objects. Soap and strong disinfectants can be used to reduce the number of viruses on surfaces. Common antiviral surface disinfectants include bleach and phenol. These chemicals disable viruses by decomposing the capsid, envelope, and genetic material. Unfortunately, these chemicals are irritating to the skin and mucous membranes, so they must be used carefully to prevent harm.

Hygiene prophylaxis is ineffective in preventing yellow fever. This disease is spread by living vectors and not by direct contact or nonliving vectors that can be sterilized. The focus has to be on preventing the spread of the virus by the mosquito or that is being stored in the bodies of alternative hosts such as monkeys. Traditional methods involve controlling mosquitoes by removing the mosquito's breeding grounds or by killing the mosquitoes with pesticides. Both methods were used effectively in the 1900s to initially control yellow fever. However, this approach is no longer feasible.

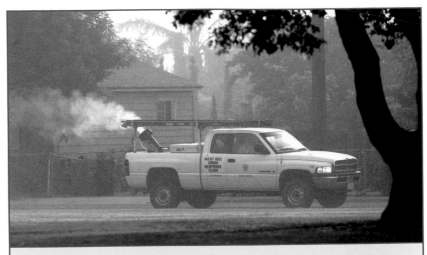

Figure 7.2 Many municipalities spread pesticides to control the mosquito populations that spread yellow fever. (© AP Images)

First, it has been seen that removing mosquito habitats disrupts the lives of other organisms that need the water and can cause severe damage to the environment. Some researchers introduced fish that selectively eat mosquitoes in an attempt to reduce the mosquito population. This also becomes ineffective because the fish either die off or adapt to eating other insects in place of the mosquitoes. Pesticides also cause problems because they poison beneficial insects as well as other organisms such as birds and fish.

One study on malaria may prove useful for controlling yellow fever. Researchers have genetically modified vector mosquitoes so they cannot transmit malaria. The virus fails to replicate in the mosquito's body and then cannot be transmitted to another host during a blood feeding. These genetically modified mosquitoes can then be released into the environment where they replicate and pass the trait to wild mosquitoes. Researchers still have to ensure that the mosquitoes last in the wild and will not cause environmental harm as a result of the genetic modification. A

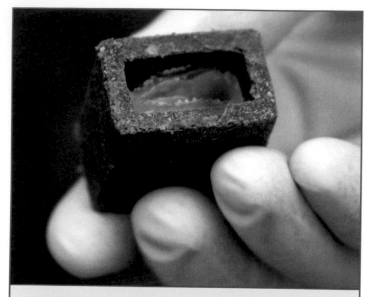

Figure 7.3 Vaccine baits such as the ones used to immunize raccoons against rabies can be used to control yellow fever in monkeys and other wild host animals. (© AP Images)

similar strategy was used to control a cattle disease in Texas caused by the screw worm fly. Male flies were exposed to radiation so they became sterile. They were then released into the environment and competed for mates with wild flies. Female flies mating the sterile males had no offspring for that mating season. Ultimately, this technique reduced the population of flies and got the disease under control.

Another future prophylactic strategy for yellow fever may involve vaccinating wild animals against yellow fever. In the 1990s, a new strategy for controlling rabies was devised, using rabies vaccine bait. Scientists discovered that wild raccoons were capable of spreading rabies to domesticated animals that then transmitted the fatal disease to humans. So, a program was developed in the United State in which rabies bait was dropped by airplanes into forests where raccoons lived. The raccoons ate the bait and then developed immunity against rabies. This program proved successful and has been expanded to control rabies in other wild animals. It is hoped that a similar strategy can be used to bait monkeys with a yellow fever vaccine. Monkeys are a reservoir for yellow fever in many countries and are the focal point for human yellow fever outbreaks.

Public health officials are currently confident that yellow fever is under control. There are regular outbreaks primarily because many people have not been vaccinated against the disease. Outbreaks typically appear in unvaccinated populations. Unfortunately, viruses are capable of adapting to new conditions and can evolve traits that thwart the best attempts at controlling them. This holds true for the yellow fever virus. Also, factors such as global climate change and water pollution may change the distribution and frequency of yellow fever worldwide. Public health officials and scientists are well aware that controlling infectious diseases is an ongoing battle. However, advances in biotechnology and medicine are making the war against yellow fever safer and more efficient.

Notes

Chapter 1

1. The New York Times Online Archives, http://query.nytimes.com/mem/archive-free/pdf?res=9401E4D8143EE63BBC40 53DFBF668383669FDE (accessed October 31, 2008).
2. P.W. Bryan, *The Papyrus Ebers* (London: Geoffrey Bles, 1930).
3. L. Debbie, "Yellow Fever and the Slave Trade: Coleridge's The Rime of the Ancient Mariner." *English Literary History* 65, no. 3 (1998): pp. 675-700.
4. R. W. Boyce, "Proof of the Endemic Origin of Yellow Fever in West Africa," *British Medical Journal* 2, no. 2605 (1910): 177.

Chapter 2

1. Centers for Disease Control and Prevention. "Yellow Fever Alert for Brazil – Updated," http://wwwn.cdc.gov/travel/contentYellowFeverBrazil.aspx (updated July 29, 2008).
2. International Committee on Taxonomy of Viruses, http://www.ictvonline.org/index.asp?bhcp=1 (accessed May 29, 2009).

Chapter 3

1. R. E. Shope, "Global Climate Change and Infectious Diseases," *Environmental Health Perspectives* 96 (1991): 171-74.
2. J. Henle, *On Miasmata and Contagia*, trans. George Rosen (Baltimore: Johns Hopkins University Press, 1938).

Chapter 4

1. F. L. Moore, G. M. Edington, and J. A. Smith, "A Clinicopathological Study of Human Yellow Fever," *Bulletin of the World Health Organization* 46 (1972): 659–67.
2. J.C. Wilson, *Infectious Diseases* (New York: Appleton, 1911).
3. Centers for Disease Control and Prevention. "Yellow Fever Prevention," http://www.cdc.gov/ncidod/dvbid/YellowFever/YF_Prevention.html (accessed May 29, 2009).

Chapter 5

1. F. G. Kilgour, "Science in the American Colonies and the Early Republic, 1664-1845," *Journal of World History* 10, no. 2 (1967): 393-415.

Chapter 6

1. H. A. Kelly, *Walter Reed and Yellow Fever* (New York: McClure, Phillips & Co, 1906).
2. J. C. Reed, A. Agramonte, and J. W. Lazear, "The Etiology of Yellow Fever —A Preliminary Note," *Proceedings of the Twenty-eighth Annual Meeting of the American Public Health Association*, October 1900.

Glossary

adenovirus—A virus that invades the upper respiratory system.

adsorption—The process of sticking onto something.

agents—A chemical or organism that carries out a particular function.

allergy—A severe immune system response to certain substances.

anthrax—A bacterial disease of cattle and humans that causes severe internal bleeding.

antibiotics—A drug that selectively kills bacteria.

antibody—An immune system chemical that attaches to foreign substances in the body.

antigen—Any substance that can produce an immune response.

antimicrobial—Something that kills microorganisms.

antiviral—A disinfectant treatment that destroys viruses.

apoptosis—A situation in which cells can program their own death using a strategy called programmed cell death.

arthropod—A large group of animals that lack a backbone and have jointed appendages and a hard outside skeleton.

attachment proteins—Viral capsid proteins that help a virus complete its life cycle.

attenuated—A vaccine term that means weakened.

bacteria—A primitive single-cell microorganism that feeds on dead matter or lives as a pathogen on animals and plants.

bacteriophage—A virus that attacks bacteria.

biotechnology—Any technology based on using the chemistry of living organisms in applications related to agriculture, food science, and medicine.

bird flu—Also known as avian influenza, it is a type of virus that harms the respiratory system of birds and can be spread to other animals.

cancer—A diseased growth or tumor caused by abnormal and uncontrolled cell division.

capsid—A viral structure that surrounds the genome.

capsomere—A subunit protein that makes up a viral capsid.

carrier—A person or animal not showing the disease but possessing the infectious agent.

case-control study—A respective epidemiology study done on a new disease.

cell—The smallest unit of life that makes up an organism.

cell membrane—A lipid and protein covering that encloses the cytoplasm of a cell.

Centers for Disease Control and Prevention—A federal organization in the United States that monitors diseases.

central nervous system—Part of the nervous system composed of the brain and spinal column.

cerebrospinal fluid—A fluid that protects the brain and spinal cord.

cervical cancer—A cancer of the female reproductive tract caused by a virus.

Clinical Surveillance Program—A program for diagnosing disease established by the National Institutes of Health.

clinical test—Medical testing done on body samples that helps determine the cause of a disease.

competent—A condition in which a vector is capable of harboring a disease organism.

contagious—The ease with which a disease can be transmitted from one person to another.

convalescence—Recovery from a disease.

Creutzfeldt-Jakob Disease (CJD)—A nervous system disease of humans caused by a prion.

crystallography—A technique that uses X-rays to determine the shapes of large molecules.

cytoplasm—Cellular material that is within the cell membrane.

dengue fever—A deadly viral disease of humans spread by mosquitoes.

deoxyribonucleic acid (DNA)—The chemical that makes up the genetic material of cells.

diagnose—To detect and identify a disease.

diagnosis—The actions needed to diagnose a disease.

disinfectant—A chemical or treatment that disables or removes microorganisms.

DNA virus—A virus with DNA as its genetic material.

domestication—The process of breeding animals for traits that serve human purposes.

double-stranded—A term used to describe nucleic acid molecules made up of two chains of nucleic acids attached side by side.

electrocardiogram—A medical procedure that measures the electrical activity of the heart.

electron—A negatively charged particle that orbits the nucleus of an atom.

electron microscope—A powerful microscope that uses electrons to magnify an object.

electrophoresis—A procedure by which molecules can be separated according to size and electrical charge as a means of identification.

encephalitis—Inflammation of the brain.

endemic—The regular presence of a disease or an infectious agent in a certain population.

endoplasmic reticulum—A structure in cells that helps manufacture proteins.

envelope—A covering on the virus that resembles a cell membrane.

enveloped virus—Viruses that possess an envelope that surrounds the capsid.

enzyme—A protein that carries out specific chemical reactions.

epidemic—The occurrence of more cases of disease than expected in a given area or among a specific group of people within a certain period of time.

epidemiologist—A scientist who studies epidemiology.

epidemiology—The study of the occurrence and frequency of disease in populations.

epithelial—Cells that form the linings of organs and body cavities.

exposure—A risk factor in the environment, such as something or a situation that brings the organism in contact with a person.

fever—Elevated body temperature caused by injury or disease.

filtering—The process of separating a mixture of substances by passing it through a filter.

flu—An infectious respiratory system disease caused by the influenza virus.

fomite—Any object or nonliving substance capable of transmitting infectious organisms.

gamete—A cell involved in sexual reproduction.

gene—A sequence of DNA that represents a fundamental unit of heredity.

genetically modified—Altering a cell's genetic material using genetic engineering.

genetic engineering—A technology used to alter the genetic material of living cells.

genetics—The study of DNA structure, function, and inheritance.

genome—The complete genetic material of an organism.

genus—A category of classification that groups one or more closely related species of organisms.

hepatitis G—A viral disease of humans that causes liver damage.

herpes—A viral disease that infects the skin and the nervous system.

host—An organism that provides resources for the survival of a parasite.

hygiene—The practice of cleanliness techniques that maintain health.

immune response—A set of reactions the body uses to attack and remove foreign substances that enter the body.

immune system—An organ system of the body that fights disease and heals the body after damage.

immunization—A process by which protection to an infectious disease or cancer is administered.

immunoglobin—An antibody.

immunoglobin G—A type of antibody found in the serum during a disease.

immunoglobulin—A protein used to battle foreign substances.

immunohistochemistry—A chemical procedure that uses antibodies to detect the presence of disease organisms.

incubation period—The time from contact with an infectious organism to the first signs or symptoms of disease.

incubator—A chamber used to grow cells or organisms under precise environmental conditions.

infectious—A disease readily spread from one organism to another.

inflammation—An immune response that produces redness, swelling, pain, and a feeling of heat that helps protect the body from infections or injury.

interference RNA—A technique that uses RNA molecules to disrupt or modify cellular processes.

interferon—A type of interleukin used to combat viral infections.

interleukin—A chemical that protects the body from viral infections.

International Committee on Taxonomy of Viruses (ICTV)—An international group of scientists that sets policies on the classification of viruses.

intoxication—To become poisoned.

intracellular—Something that takes place inside a cell.

in vitro—Refers to culturing organisms or conducting experiments under laboratory conditions.

jaundice—A liver ailment characterized by yellowing of the skin.

kidney dialysis—A medical treatment using a machine that replaces the function of the kidneys.

latent period—The time between the measurable onset of disease and detection of the disease.

leprosy—A infectious bacterial disease that damages bones, skin, and the nervous system.

life cycle—The time period from birth to death of an organism.

lysis—The breakdown and subsequent death of a cell.

mad cow disease—A brain disease of cattle caused by prions.

malaria—A disease that is spread by mosquitoes and is caused by a protist called *Plasmodium.*

malnourished—A person suffering from malnutrition.

malnutrition—A disease condition caused by a lack of certain nutrients in the diet.

mammal—An animal that possesses fur and feeds milk to its young.

Management Sciences for Health (MSH)—A non-profit group the works to improve health care management.

maturation phase—The stage of viral infection in which new viruses are assembled.

metabolism—A series of chemical reactions that carry out the functions of a cell and an organism.

microbiologist—A person who studies microscopic organisms and cell structures.

microorganism—Any microscopic living organism such as algae, bacteria, fungi, and protists.

microscope—An instrument that uses a combination of lenses or mirrors to produce magnified images of very small objects.

molecule—The name given to a chemical made up of two or more atoms.

morbidity—Any illness resulting from a disease.

mortality—A measure of the occurrence of death from a disease in a particular population of people during a particular period of time.

mucus—A thick secretion produced in cells lining the digestive and respiratory systems.

mutation—A genetic change that occurs in an organism.

National Institutes of Health—A governmental agency that oversees health issues and medical research.

nausea—The feeling of wanting to throw up or vomit.

negative-sense RNA—A reversed copy of the functional RNA.

neurotropic—Refers to a disease organism that attacks the brain or nervous system.

nucleic acid—A complex molecule associated with the structure and function of genetic material. DNA and RNA are composed of nucleic acids.

nucleocapsid—An inner capsid that directly surrounds the viral genome.

nucleotide—A nucleic acid attached in a chain to other nucleic acids.

nucleus—A structure in eukaryotic cells that contains the genetic material.

organ—A specialized structure in an organism that carries out particular body functions.

outbreak—The sudden, violent, spontaneous occurrence of a disease.

pandemic—A widespread disease.

parasite—An organism that lives in or on the living tissue of a host organism at the expense of that host.

parasitic—A condition in which an organism lives in or on the living tissue of a host organism at the expense of that host.

parenteral—Refers to a drug given by injection.

particle—A name given to viruses and related organisms that do not possess the major properties of life.

passive vaccine—An immunoglobin treatment that enhances the immune system for the duration of a disease

pathogen—An organism that causes disease.

penetration—The action of entering into or through something.

poliomyelitis—A viral disease that affects the nervous system.

polymerase chain reaction (PCR)—A biotechnology procedure for making multiple copies of genetic material from very small samples.

positive-sense RNA—A type of RNA that contains genetic information in a conventional format.

presumptive diagnosis—The probable diagnosis of a disease using a physical examination.

primate—A category of mammals that includes monkeys, apes, and humans.

prion—An infectious particle composed of protein.

prognosis—A prediction of the course and outcome of the disease condition.

promoter—A piece of DNA that facilitates the expression of a gene.

prophylactic—Strategies used to prevent the spread of disease.

prospective epidemiology—A technique used to determine whether a disease may happen in a person or a population in the future.

protein—A complex molecule made up of amino acids that are needed for cell structure and function.

protist—A microscopic organism related to both animals and plants.

pyrogen—A substance that causes the elevation of body temperature.

rabies—A viral disease that affects the nervous system of many types of mammals.

receptor—A protein that binds to specific types of chemicals.

release phase—The final stage of viral infection in which new viruses are released from the cell.

remedy—A treatment used to cure or treat an ailment.

remission—The state of absence of disease activity.

repressor proteins—Viral proteins that control cell function during a virus's replication.

retrospective epidemiology—Investigation of a disease after it has already happened.

ribonucleic acid (RNA)—A chemical similar to DNA, it is a nucleic acid involved in the production of proteins.

risk factor—A term explaining the circumstances that cause a person to develop a disease.

RNA virus—A virus with RNA as its genetic material.

St. Louis encephalitis—A viral disease of humans that damages the brain and spinal cord.

saliva—A fluid produced by the salivary glands.

salivary gland—A digestive gland found in the mouths of many organisms.

seizure—Uncontrolled jerking movements of the body.

self-assembling—The ability of a chemical to form complex structures on their own accord by attaching to each other or to other chemicals.

serum—The liquid portion of blood.

sign—Any evidence of the presence of a disease that can be measured or detected.

single-stranded—A term used to describe nucleic acid molecules made up of only one chain.

sleeping sickness—A disease that is spread by biting flies and is caused by protists called trypanosomes.

smallpox—A deadly viral disease of humans that causes scarring of the skin and internal organs.

symptom—Evidence of a disease as perceived by the patient.

syndrome—A disease condition that affects many body organs.

therapy—A chemical treatment or procedure used as a medical cure for disease.

tissue—A group of similar cells that work together to carry out a particular function.

titer—A unit used to measure the amount of a virus in a host's body.

transmission—The passing of a disease organism from an infected organism to one that is not infected with the disease.

treatment—A medical strategy used for alleviating disease.

tuberculosis—A bacterial disease that affects the lungs and bones.

uncoating—A stage of viral infection in which the capsid is removed from the virus.

undernourished—A person not receiving enough food to be healthy.

United Nations—An independent organization of nations formed in 1945 to promote international peace and security.

United States Food and Drug Administration—This government agency is a branch of the Department of Health and Human Services. It works on health and policy issues for cosmetics, drugs, food, and medical treatments.

vaccination—The process by which a person's immune system is induced to develop protection from a particular disease.

vector—An organism or object that passes a disease between people or other organisms.

vector assisted transmission—Spread of a disease by a vector.

vertebrate—An animal with a backbone and internal skeleton.

viral—A term that refers to a virus.

viral hemorrhagic fever (VHF)—A group of viral diseases noted for their ability to damage many body organs.

viricide—A substance that disables viruses.

viroid—An organism composed of circular piece of infectious RNA.

virology—The scientific investigation of viruses and viral diseases.

virulent—Something that is extremely infectious or poisonous.

virus—A small particle that infects cells.

virusoid—An organism composed of simple infectious RNA.

vomiting—The release of stomach contents through the mouth.

West Nile disease—A viral disease of humans that damages the membranes of the brain and the nervous system.

white blood cell—A group of blood cells involved in the immune response.

World Health Organization—A branch of the United Nations that monitors diseases globally.

yellow fever—A serious viral disease spread by mosquitoes.

zoonotic—A disease that can be spread from animals to humans.

Further Resources

Books

Alberts, B., J. Lewis, M. Raff, A. Johnson, and K. Roberts. *Molecular Biology of the Cell.* London: Taylor & Francis, 2002.

Alcamo, I. E. *DNA Technology: The Awesome Skill.* Philadelphia: Elsevier Science & Technology Books, 2000.

Banatvala, J., and C. Peckham. R*ubella Viruses, Volume 15 (Perspectives in Medical Virology).* Amsterdam: Elsevier Science, 2007.

Bauman R., E. Machunis-Masuoka, and I. R. Tizard. *Microbiology.* San Francisco: Pearson Education, 2004.

Bynum, W. F., and R. Porter, eds. *Companion Encyclopedia of the History of Medicine.* London: Routledge, 1993.

Carter, J., and V. Saunders. *Virology: Principles and Applications.* New York: John Wiley and Sons, 2007.

Corlett, W. T. *A Treatise On The Acute, Infectious Exanthemata; Including Variola, Rubeola, Scarlatina, Rubella, Varicella and Vaccinia.* Whitefish, Mont.: Kessinger Publishing, 2007.

Council for International Organizations of Medical Sciences (CIOMS) in collaboration with the World Health Organization. *International Ethical Guidelines for Biomedical Research Involving Human Subjects.* Geneva: CIOMS and WHO, 1993.

Diamond, J. *Guns, Germs and Steel: The Fates of Human Societies.* New York: Norton, W. W. & Company, 1999.

Kaufman. S. R. *The Healer's Tale.* Madison: The University of Wisconsin Press, 1993.

Kelly, H. A. *Walter Reed and Yellow Fever.* New York: McLure, Phillips, 1907.

Levine, R. J. "Research in Emergency Situations the Role of Deferred Consent." *Journal of the American Medical Association* 273, no. 16: 1300–02.

Porter, R., ed. *Cambridge Illustrated History of Medicine.* Cambridge, Mass.: Cambridge University Press, 1996.

Powell, J. H., K. R. Foster, and A. C. Toogood. *Bring Out Your Dead: The Great Plague of Yellow Fever in Philadelphia in 1793.* Philadelphia: University of Pennsylvania Press, 1993.

Ratner, M. A., and D. Ratner. *Nanotechnology: A Gentle Introduction to the Next Big Idea.* Upper Saddle River, N.J.: Prentice Hall, 2002.

Shmaefsky, B. R. *Applied Anatomy and Physiology: A Case Study Approach.* St. Paul, Minn.: EMC/Paradigm, 2007.

Shmaefsky, B. R. *Biotechnology 101 (Science 101 series).* Westport, Conn.: Greenwood Press, 2006.

Shmaefsky, B. R. *Medicine in the News (Science News Flash).* New York: Chelsea House Publications, 2007.

Shorter, E. *The Health Century.* New York: Doubleday, 1987.

Travers, B., ed. *Medical Discoveries: Medical Breakthroughs and the People Who Developed Them.* Volumes 1–3. Farmington Hills, Mich.: UXL Publishing, 1997.

Zuckerman, J. N. *Principles and Practices of Travel Medicine.* New York: John Wiley and Sons, 2001.

Web Sites

Biotechnology Industries Organization
http://www.bio.org

Centers for Disease Control & Prevention – Yellow Fever
http://www.cdc.gov/ncidod/dvbid/yellowfever

Cold Spring Harbor Laboratory
http://www.cshl.org

HealthLink. Medical College of Wisconsin.
http://healthlink.mcw.edu

International Committee on Taxonomy of Viruses – Yellow Fever
http://phene.cpmc.columbia.edu/ICTVdB/00.026.0.01.001.htm

Martin Memorial Health System
http://www.mmhs.com

Mayo Clinic.com
http://www.mayoclinic.com

Medline Plus
(U.S. National Library of Medicine and the National Institutes of Health)
http://www.medlineplus.gov

Microbiology Bytes
http://www.microbiologybytes.com/introduction/index.html

National Library of Medicine
http://www.nlm.nih.gov

Virology Journal
http://www.virology.net

World Health Organization – Yellow Fever
http://www.who.int/topics/yellow_fever/en

Index

climate, tropical, 36–37, 45, 47–48, 64, 81, 84
climate change, 36, 95
Clinical Surveillance Program (CSP), 52, 97
clinical tests, 52, 54–58, 97
clothing, 62
Columbus, Christopher, 45
commerce, in disease transmission, 37–38, 48–49, 64, 69, 74, 76
communicable diseases
  caused by microorganisms, 6, 9–10
  control of, 6–7
  deaths caused by, 6, 47–49, 56
competency, vector, 38–39, 98
Congo, Democratic Republic of, 68, 69
contagious disease, 44, 98
containment, 61, 70
control, 88–95. *See also* mosquito control; prevention
  of communicable diseases, 6–7
  difficulty of, 7, 11, 66, 95
  future of, 88–95
  prophylactic strategies of, 92–95
  public perceptions of, 79–81
  of smallpox, 74–76
  of vectors, 11, 19, 20, 47, 54, 60, 66
  of viral life cycle, 88–92
  of yellow fever, 60–66, 92–95
convalescence, 56, 60, 98
coup de barre, 44
cowpox, 74
Creutzfeldt-Jakob Disease (CJD), 6, 23, 98
crystallography, 23, 98

CSP. *See* Clinical Surveillance Program
Cuba, 15, 19, 82
cytoplasm, 31, 39, 98

DDT, 60
deaths. *See* mortality
defective viruses, 32
dengue fever, 34, 36, 53, 98
deoxyribonucleic acid. *See* DNA
developing world
  access to health care in, 7, 46, 47–49
  communicable diseases in, 6–7, 47
diagnosis
  definition of, 51, 98
  difficulty of, 50
  presumptive, 51–52, 103
  of yellow fever, 12, 50–58
dichloro-diphenyl-trichloroethane (DDT), 60
diet, 48
direct transmission, 10
disabled viruses. *See* vaccine(s)
disabling communicable diseases, 6, 7
disinfectants, 88, 98
DNA, 24–25, 28, 74, 98
DNA viruses
  definition of, 25, 99
  replication of, 25, 29, 30–33, 39–41
  structure of, 25, 26
domestic animals, 71, 74, 76, 99
double-stranded molecules, 25, 26, 29, 99
drugs. *See also specific types of drugs*
  effectiveness of, 7
  resistance to, 6, 7, 95
  in treatment of yellow fever, 59–60, 91

Ebola, 11, 37, 68–70
eclipse phase, 31
economic costs, 6, 76, 78–79
education, 7, 20, 73
eggs
  mosquito, 39
  in vaccine development, 62, 65, 89
Egypt, 13, 20–21
EKG. *See* electrocardiogram
electrocardiogram (EKG), 55, 99
electron(s), 99
electron microscopes, 22, 99
electrophoresis, 57, 99
ELISA. *See* enzyme-linked immunosorbent assay
emerging diseases, 6, 76
encephalitis, 34, 65, 99, 104
endemic diseases, 36, 37, 44, 45, 47, 99
endoplasmic reticulum, 41, 99
England, 70
envelope(s), definition of, 28, 99
enveloped viruses
  definition of, 28, 99
  life cycle of, 31, 33
  replication of, 39–41
  smallpox as, 74
  structure of, 28, 34–35
environment
  climate change in, 36
  and mosquitoes, 11, 20, 21, 37, 84
  pesticides in, 60, 92–93
  risk factors in, 44, 49, 56–57, 62
  in transmission of yellow fever, 14, 20, 36–37
  in viral genome damage, 24–25
  in viral life cycle, 29–30
enzyme-linked immunosorbent assay (ELISA), 57–58

About the Author

Dr. Brian Shmaefsky is a professor of biology and service learning coordinator at Lone Star College, Kingwood, near Houston, Texas. He completed his undergraduate studies in biology at Brooklyn College in New York and completed his graduate studies at Southern Illinois University at Edwardsville and at the University of Illinois. His research emphasis is in environmental physiology. Dr. Shmaefsky has many publications on science education, some appearing in *American Biology Teacher* and the *Journal of College Science Teaching*. He also has written books and technical articles on biotechnology and human diseases. Dr. Shmaefsky is also the author of an anatomy and physiology textbook. He is very active serving on local and international environmental awareness and policy committees. He has two children, Kathleen and Timothy, and lives in Kingwood, Texas, with his two dogs and a guinea pig.

About the Consulting Editor

Hilary Babcock, M.D., M.P.H., is an assistant professor of medicine at Washington University School of Medicine and Medical Director of Occupational Health for Barnes-Jewish Hospital and St. Louis Children's Hospital. She received her undergraduate degree from Brown University and her M.D. from the University of Texas Southwestern Medical Center at Dallas. After completing her residency, chief residency, and infectious disease fellowship at Barnes-Jewish Hospital, she joined the faculty of the Infectious Disease division. She completed an M.P.H. in Public Health from St. Louis University School of Public Health in 2006. She has lectured, taught, and written extensively about infectious diseases, their treatment, and their prevention. She is a member of numerous medical associations and is board certified in infectious disease. She lives in St. Louis, Missouri.